Home Care Nursing Services

Doris M. Modly, RN, PhD, FAAN, is Professor of Nursing and Director of International Health Programs at the Frances Payne Bolton School of Nursing, Case Western Reserve University (CWRU) in Cleveland, Ohio. She also directs the school's World Health Organization (WHO) Collaborating Center for Research and Clinical Training in Home Care Nursing. Dr. Modly earned her bachelor's, master's and doctoral degrees in nursing from CWRU, as well as a master's degree in medical anthropology. Among many other international accomplishments, Dr. Modly has worked to develop home care conferences, seminars and exchange programs in Korea, Thailand, and Hungary. Her efforts to introduce a university-based nursing program in Hungary earned Dr. Modly the Officers Cross of the Order of Merit of the Republic of Hungary. She has also facilitated an exchange program allowing Hungarian students and faculty to observe the home care program at CWRU and has played an essential role in the establishment of the WHO Collaborating Center in Budapest. This important work has led to her recently receiving the 1997 Fulbright Fellowship to continue the projects she has initiated in Hungary on a more concentrated scale from January through June of 1997.

Renzo Zanotti, RN, AFD, PhD, is Professor of Nursing at Padua University, Italy. He is Director of the International Institute of Nursing Research (ISIR), Padua, and Director of the European Association for Nursing Diagnosis, Activities and Outcomes (ACENDIO). He is an active researcher and has authored books and scientific articles on nursing care in the home setting. He consults on home care development for many Italian local health agencies.

Dott. Piera Poletti is President of the Center for Research and Education (CEREF) based in Padua, Italy. She teaches and consults in continuing education in nursing for many hospitals and community agencies. She is a leading consultant in projects of quality improvement in health care settings for Italian regional and local agencies. She has authored books and articles based on her research. Her activity in developing international networks has encouraged systematic collaborative research projects.

Joyce J. Fitzpatrick, PhD, is the Elizabeth Brooks Ford Professor and Dean of the Frances Payne Bolton School of Nursing, Case Western Reserve University. She is editor of the *Annual Review of Nursing Research* series, now in its fifteenth volume.

Home Care Nursing Services

International Lessons

Doris Modly
Renzo Zanotti
Piera Poletti
Joyce J. Fitzpatrick

Editors

 Springer Publishing Company

Springer Publishing Company, Inc.
536 Broadway
New York, NY 10012-3955

Cover design by Margaret Dunin
Production Editor: Jeanne Libby

97 98 99 00 01 / 5 4 3 2 1

Library of Congress Cataloging-in-Publication Data

Developing home care nursing services : international lessons / Doris
    Modly . . . [et al.], editors.
        p.   cm.
    Includes index.
    ISBN 0-8261-9600-4
    1. Home care services.   2. Home care services—Administration.
    I. Modly, Doris Matherny.
    [DNLM: 1. Home Care Services—organization & administration. WY
    115 D489   1997]
    RA645.3.D48   1997
    362.1'4—dc21
    DNLM/DLC
    for Library of Congress   96-53472
                                                                          CIP

Printed in the United States of America

Contents

Contents

Introduction

This book presents a future perspective on health care, as care moves from hospitals into the home and the community. In 1995, the editors organized an international conference, held in Padua and Venice, Italy, attended by health care professionals from more than 30 countries; the conference was focused on home care throughout the world. As a result of the conference, the organizers believed that it was important to capture highlights of the home care developments worldwide. This book is the result of these continuing efforts.

Worldwide home care and community-based services are considered the foundation of health for all in the future. Two main factors support this common opinion: (a) the costs; and (b) the possibility for the patient to remain in her or his life environment. Therefore, in almost all countries, services have been developed in the last few years. However, there have been relatively few forums for people involved in the field to learn from others' experiences. We aim to provide the readers with a general framework to approach the issue and gain knowledge from different experiences.

The content describes home care service organizations and nursing clinical practice, using examples from countries of four continents. Quality improvement, cost of home care, education, and nursing research in the field also are discussed. The need to produce scientific knowledge in home care is today perceived by many. However, there has not been enough research produced in this area. A larger investment in home care research has to be stimulated in the near future. Because home care services are so much affected by the local culture, cross-cultural research projects are recommended in this field.

In Section 4, the text contains chapters by authors from many countries. Authors discuss aspects of home care in their country. Each provides a glimpse of home care clinical and/or organizational delivery system particular to a country. The views presented are not expected to provide a comprehensive overview of home care globally, but rather are reflections of the issues confronting clinicians and health care administrators.

Most of all this book represents international lessons in home care, so that across the globe health professionals can learn from each other. Some chapters include case studies focusing on selected patient/client needs and on nursing interventions that include family and informal caregivers. This book can also guide curriculum planners in the process of redesigning nursing curricula to meet the learning needs of nurses in the future. This is particularly relevant as faculty members are designing new programs and new courses in home care.

An overview of the chapters is as follows:

Fitzpatrick introduces the book by describing the trends of nursing from a worldwide perspective.

Zanotti gives a general overview of caring at home. He describes the uniqueness of nursing services delivered in the home, stressing the implication for the nurse, client, and family. Moreover, he discusses the role and potentials of the different resources that can be activated in the home setting.

Worldwide issues in organizing home-based health care are discussed by Modly in the section on an international overview of home care. Selected problems and country-specific solutions are given as examples.

Martinson bases her chapter on her extensive experience with home-based care of dying children both in the United States and abroad. The importance of home care for children is poignantly presented.

Munodawafa and McDonald collaborated on the chapter pertaining to community-based care of patients suffering from acquired immunodeficiency syndrome (AIDS) in Zimbabwe. The importance of family support is stressed.

Geys describes the complex system of home care delivery in Belgium. He explains how the system has developed and the current available services.

Moers describes the development of the home care in Germany from a historical and conceptual perspective. A clear distinction is made between health care and social support care.

The Dutch home care services, their history, and trends are explained in Kerkstra's chapter.

A description of the home care services in Finland is offered in Vehviläinen-Julkunen's chapter. She also discusses research findings and future developments.

Two main features of the United Kingdom home care services are presented in the book. Wagner describes the clients and services offered by the "Hospital-at-Home." She also presents examples of this approach to provide the reader with a complete understanding of the difference from traditional care delivered at home. Orr outlines the role of the health visitor in the United Kingdom, a nurse specialist who not just intervenes when necessary, but monitors the population needs and activates many different strategies to promote the well-being of the population.

Balogh and Modly discuss an experimental program of home-based care of the hemiplegic patient in a specific district in Budapest, Hungary, where the number of stroke victims is rather significant, and the need for home-based rehabilitation services is high.

Changes in societal norms and cultural precedence bring with them new needs for care of the old and ill in Korea as well. Managing the care of elders through home care nurses is discussed by Lee and associates.

Cunico describes the history of home care psychiatric services in Italy. She explores the new philosophy of the services and the main steps in their implementation. In addition, the role of the nurse working in the field is described as well as the new trends in patient treatments.

A clear picture of the psychiatric home nurse's activity is provided by Proehl and Berila. They describe and comment on three cases of patients successfully treated at home. The nurse's therapeutic activities are described and placed into a broader scientific framework.

An overview of home and community care in Australia is given in Schultz's chapter. She also describes the role of the primary caregivers, and their feelings and needs. The necessity to equip them with skills and insights is stressed, and an example of a special program is provided.

Pitorak describes hospice services as a kind of home-based nursing care provided for the terminally ill. Hospice care has become a trend in health care in the United States as well as worldwide.

The most innovative component of home nursing is the increasing use of highly technical aids and instruments in the provision of home-based care. Chulay confirms this in her chapter concerning the use of the technology used in the home nursing care setting.

Quality improvement is the core of Marrelli's chapter. She describes the quality improvement process, and presents quality's indicators and the commonalities that support quality in home care nursing, transcending the diversity of geographics, cultures, and economic policies.

Poletti outlines the role of basic continuing education. She describes strategies, contents, and didactic methodologies to be used in preparing professionals who work in the home care setting.

Barkauskas's review of home care nursing research highlights three areas: studies pertaining to the needs of individuals for home care, evaluations of the effectiveness and efficiency of home care, and descriptions of home health providers. The importance of future research and the development of a common taxonomy for nursing diagnosis and interventions are also discussed.

It is our expectation that this book will serve as a platform for future conferences, research projects, and short training courses focused on home care nursing. Much remains to be done to prepare and position nurses and other health care workers so that they best meet the needs of patients, families, and communities through this new home care emphasis.

Doris M. Modly
Renzo Zanotti
Piera Poletti
Joyce J. Fitzpatrick

Contributors

Zoltán Balogh, RN, BScN, Lecturer, Hajnal Imre University, Department of Nursing, Budapest, Hungary

Violet H. Barkauskas, RN, PhD, FAAN, Associate Professor, Associate Dean for Organizational Planning & Support, School of Nursing, The University of Michigan, Ann Arbor, MI

Rose-Anne M. Berila, RN, MSN, Psychiatric Nursing, Cleveland Clinic Foundation, Cleveland, OH

Marianne Chulay, RN, DNSc, FAAN, Director, Nursing Research and Clinical Practice, Moses Cone Health System, Greensboro, NC

June Clark, RN, DBE, PhD, RHV, FRCN, Professor, School of Nursing, Middlesex University, Enfield, United Kingdom

AFD Dott. Laura Cunico, Professor of Psychiatric Nursing, University of Padua, Padua, Italy

Joyce J. Fitzpatrick, RN, MBA, PhD, FAAN, Professor and Dean of Nursing, FPB School of Nursing, Case Western Reserve University, Cleveland, OH

Ludo Geys, RN, MScN, Head of the Nursing Department, White & Yellow Cross of Belgium, Brussels, Belgium

Ae-Ran Hwang, RN, PhD, Associate Professor, College of Nursing, Yonsei University, Seoul, Korea

Ada Kerkstra, PhD, Coordinator of Nursing Research, Netherlands Institute of Primary Health Care (NIVEL), Utrecht, The Netherlands

Hea-Young Kim, RN, BSN, Division of Home Care Nursing Department, Yonsei University, Medical Center, Seoul, Korea

HaeOk Lee, RN, DNS, Assistant Professor, FPB School of Nursing, Case Western Reserve University, Cleveland, OH

Tina M. Marrelli, MA, BSN, RNC, Consultant, T. M. Marrelli and Associates, Westerville, OH

Ida M. Martinson, RN, PhD, FAAN, Chair of Nursing, Head of Department of Health Sciences, The Hong Kong Polytechnic University, Hung Hom Kowloon, Hong Kong

Patricia E. McDonald, RN, PhD, Assistant Professor, FPB School of Nursing, Case Western Reserve University, Cleveland, OH

Doris M. Modly, RN, MA, PhD, FAAN, Professor and Director, International Health Program and World Health Organization Collaborating Center for Nursing, Case Western Reserve University, Cleveland, OH

Martin Moers, RN, PhD, Professor of Nursing, Fachhochschule Osnabruek, Osnabrueck, Germany

Auxilia Munodawafa, RN, SCM, DNA, ANP, MSN, Lecturer, University of Zimbabwe, Harare, Zimbabwe

Jean A. Orr, BA, Msc, RGN, RHV, HV TUT CERT, Professor and Director, School of Nursing, Queen's University of Belfast, Belfast, United Kingdom

Elizabeth Ford Pitorak, RN, MSN, CRNH, Hospice Coordinator, Hospice of the Western Reserve, Cleveland, OH

Dott. Piera Poletti, Director of CEREF, Center of Nursing Research and Education, Padua, Italy

Katherine Jubell Proehl, RN, ND, Lecturer, FPB School of Nursing, Case Western Reserve, Cleveland, OH

Cynthia L. Schultz, BA (Hons), PhD, MAPS, Sr. Lecturer, School of Behavioral Health Sciences, La Trobe University, Bundoora, Victoria, Australia

Katri Vehvilainen-Julkunen, RN, PhD, Professor, University of Kuopio, Department of Nursing, Kuopio, Finland

Violet Wagner, BA, SRN, RSCN, HV, Cert., Director of Nursing, South Essex Health Authority, Billerisay, Essex, United Kingdom

Renzo Zanotti, RN, AFD, PhD, Professor of Nursing, University of Padua, Padua, Italy

PART I

Home Care Nursing from an International Perspective

CHAPTER 1

Home Care Nursing: Uniqueness and Diversity

Renzo Zanotti

Nursing is a discipline that deals with phenomena within the human field of health. Other disciplines in the same field share many phenomena with nursing, sometimes competing, sometimes collaborating, often overlapping each other. Nursing as an integrating discipline struggles to define and defend its own domain, its cultural identity. The history of nursing is a story of compassion; empathy; benevolence; and, recently, science. Thus, it is also a story of contradictions between humanity and technical skills, between therapeutic relationships and detachment. Actually, all these contradictions are still present in the nursing culture and nurse's clinical activity. However, despite the presence of so many contrasts and the long history of changes, the nursing discipline continues with a clear, unchanged social mission that encompasses institutionalism, nationalism, and cultural diversities. The mission remains that of helping persons with health alterations, or at risk of such, to deal with them; to compensate; to adapt; to change; or, eventually, just to die. In each step, the nursing culture leads its carrier to consider the person's problem as a whole and prevents the individual from breaking the link between person and health/disease. As a consequence, we can say that a nurse provides care to the person with health alterations (or at risk of such) and does not cure the disease of the person. In carrying out some activities, nursing can look like medicine, but its social mission, and, therefore, its disciplinary culture, have to be different to guarantee the maximum benefit for society.

It is the uniqueness of cultural diversity and the focus of its disciplinary perspective that makes a nurse a nurse at home, in a hospital, or wherever he or she is providing care.

CARING AT HOME

In the complex pattern of nursing activities, the environment plays an important role, emphasizing some of the caregiver's features and obscuring others. Home is part of the client's identity. It is a milieu interacting with the nurse–patient relationship and challenging the nurse individually, person to person. Caring at the patient's home forces the nurse to face his or her mission unprotected, exposed, having to act professionally without the hospital resource redundancy. Often alone, the nurse at the patient's home has no colleagues in whom to find support and with whom to share the patient's expectancies. Exposed to unpredictable risks, but also free to be a health professional in front of his or her client, the nurse displays his or her diversity and uniqueness. In home care, the nurse has to be able and willing to carry out different informal roles, such as counselor and patient's confidant, teacher and family's observer, with a large range of styles, from assertive to authoritarian, but always beneficial to the client and the family. There is a unique mandate for the nurse taking care at home: to keep his or her attention focused beyond and despite the disease, and, meanwhile, because of the disease (or the risk of it). Carrying out this professional mandate is more energy demanding than just simply playing a technical role; it requires commitment and endurance each time the nurse passes through the door of a patient's home. The home care nurse has a commitment to be helpful to the patient and to show endurance in being an activating stimulus, not just an occasional presence.

MULTIPLICITY OF PROFESSIONAL INTERVENTIONS

Many disciplinary perspectives can be used and integrated in caring for the patient at home: psychological, sociological, and biomedical. Each one of these perspectives provide important contributions and different perspectives from which to view the patient or the family, with more comprehension and potentialities for therapeutic support. Today, the health system's organization is so developed that a patient often has a multitude of professionals available: psychologist, community nurse, physical therapist, social worker, occupational activity leader, domestic helper, general practitioner, clinical specialist, and many others. However, so many different professional perspectives and activities can be disconnected, operating out of a common therapeutic plan, but leading toward a less beneficial result for the patient. Concomitant different professional interventions can be required by the patient's health status, other members of the family, or an overlapping of situations and events, such as sickness and injuries. Family can be affected as a whole by professionals' attitudes, therapeutic prescriptions, and activities carried out when intervening at home. Thus, uncertainty, mistrust, or noncompliance can arise inside the family.

To prevent potential conflicts or misunderstandings within the family, a nurse has to be able to communicate using a language that is most understandable by other professionals. Moreover, he or she must be able to function as an integrator of different therapeutic perspectives, making them understandable for the patient and the family.

MULTIPLICITY OF NEEDS TO ASSESS

Evaluation of a patient's needs at home is a process requiring a three-dimensional assessment: (a) biophysical functionality, (b) availability of social support, and (c) psychological attitude toward self-caring (see Figure 1.1). *Biophysical functionality* is a dimension referring to a person's ill health in terms of biological status and physical capacity to perform daily life activities; its assessment requires consideration of the potential for patient or family's autonomy and limitations in type and number of self-caring activities. This dimension sets the stage for realistic goals in planning self-care activities or in defining programs for the patient's physical rehabilitation. Technically, the assessment of patient's biophysical functions requires a trained nurse, skilled in checking the patient's performances and interpreting different readings, but also able to integrate different typologies of data, such as laboratory data, physician's notes, and physical therapist's instructions, all in a meaningful synthesis.

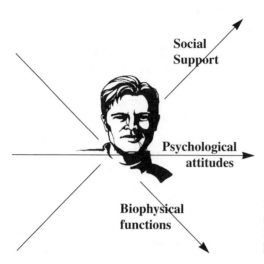

Figure 1.1 Three-dimensional assessment of the patient at home. Each axis represents a factor that has to be considered by a nurse.

Availability of social support refers to the relationships with institutions, individuals, and family members that actually or potentially are, in some ways, care providers for the patient. The assessment of this dimension requires the nurse to assess the social environment surrounding the patient, and his or her social network in particular, considering the patient's significant others, and also pattern, health, and cohesiveness of the family. Social support is a complex, multifactor dimension. An important factor that has to be carefully considered is the patient's financial status. From a nursing perspective, this means not to underestimate the patient or family's difficulties in accessing resources. Sometimes, financial distress is the main reason people do not carry out therapeutic prescriptions or even do not ask for nursing support. To assess the patient's economic status is not always an easy task. Looking at the house, furniture, and clothing, one can be fooled because they may reflect the past and not the patient's current economic condition.

Psychological attitudes refers to the psychological dimension of the patient. In this dimension, elements like self-esteem, personal commitment, and goal orientation are important factors, but other elements also need to be carefully evaluated. Personal values and beliefs, culture, and personal experiences of well-being and sickness are important in making the person more or less able to cope with the situation.

A nurse has to be a carrier of a culture focused on promoting the patient's independence in maintaining and regaining his or her autonomy. A culture focused on the patient's independence can provide perspectives, guidelines, and methods for nurses in making decisions in their daily caring activities and in coordinating interdisciplinary efforts to provide the most comprehensive support and caring for patients at home.

MULTIPLICITY OF CLINICAL SITUATIONS

Caring for people at home provides a variety of challenging situations for nurses, asking for promptness, flexibility, and confidence in their professional knowledge. There are complex clinical cases in which psychological, economic, and physical difficulties are inextricably linked. Within the variety of clinical situations, the most frequent ones requiring nursing interventions are the following:

- Terminal patients or those with progressive debilitating diseases, such as multiple sclerosis, arthritis and rheumatism, and cardiac and pulmonary diseases
- Elderly persons with limited autonomy, limited economic resources, or unsanitary or unsafe living conditions
- Patients with disabling surgical sequelae, seriously affecting self-image and social relationships, or with a high demand of therapeutic activity
- Patients who live alone with limited functional autonomy, often with fear of isolation and abandonment, and those who are widowed, depressed, or neglected
- Patients with mental health alterations

Most often these subjects are characterized by low income that causes them frustration, prevents relocation to better places, and promotes social isolation.

Nurses may realize how important it is to engage patients and families in their own social milieu effectively. It is important for the nurse to have knowledge and good training in communication techniques so that he or she can switch promptly from a dialogic to a more directive relational style when it is required for the patient's best benefit. However, even the best methodology cannot make a professional be a true nurse if he or she is not able to remain focused on the patient's autonomy, and avoid making the patient dependent on the nurse's action and knowledge.

Developing a trusting relationship has to be the first commitment for the nurse and patient to provide and receive the benefits of home care. Nurses have to trust that patients have the capacity to express their needs, and because the goal of home care is to facilitate patient independence, trust becomes an essential component of that goal (Trojan & Lange, 1993). Forming trusting relationships is particularly important when dealing with elderly people who have complex health problems, few financial resources, lower education levels, and little social support. These patients can be considered difficult or labeled as noncompliant because the nurse does not understand their reasons and behaviors, or the factors they face daily to survive. In the meantime, nurses have to be confident and trust their own skills. Patients also indicated that they had increased trust in their own skills, such as dressing changes and decision making after having contact with the nurse (Trojan & Lange, 1993). Thus, nurses' attitudes or perceptions of patients can deeply affect the type of care patients receive as well as the patients' perceptions of themselves (Solomon, 1982). Heller, Bausell, and Ninos (1994) determined that nurses with negative attitudes toward the elderly view care of the elderly as primarily custodial, whereas nurses with more positive attitudes are concerned with rehabilitation.

Nurses' attitudes are, therefore, vividly perceived by the patients. Subjects described noncaring nurses as not taking the time to listen to patients, being in a hurry, just doing a job, and being rough and belittling (Rieman, 1986). Conversely, when nurses act professionally and are personally committed, they make the patient feel safe and protected, and educated in self-care (Cronin & Harrison, 1988).

RESOURCES FOR HOME CARE

The modern development of home care systems and the much higher attention that it is getting because of economic reasons make it possible now to consider a larger variety of resources in terms of institutions, facilities, and services provided by local health and community systems. Some of these services are devoted to providing a shelter, such as boarding houses, rest homes, and temporary accommodation programs. Other services can provide financial help for needy, cultural services for elderly, or help with housework. Though these services seem to be far from a typical nurse's activity, they must be carefully considered because (a) a nurse is often interacting with them and (b) a nurse can activate their intervention or support the need for their intervention. For instance, accommodation assistance can be important for elderly who live in unsafe homes or disabled who live far from needed services. Providing them an appropriate home in a social organized environment can make elderly people more independent, reducing the risk for injuries, isolation, and depression.

The great shift in the social economy in the last 30 years has determined, in many countries, waves of emigration toward other nations or, inside a country, from agriculture to industry. This revolution in the economy, in some countries, is a cause for a new kind of separation between generations, in terms that older people remained in their traditional places while the younger people left. When operating in these areas, nurses have to consider that the community is mostly made by elderly persons or only a few older people who could not accept leaving their ancestral home. Caring for these people requires that a nurse be much more knowledgeable about resources within the community than what is required for similar cases in a more organized social context. For instance, a nurse who is caring for an elderly patient, mostly alone and understimulated, must know what the community offers in terms of public libraries; support groups; and cultural, social, and financial initiatives for the elderly. A nurse can be a resources activator, an adviser, and a stimulus for his or her patient to make the patient willing to use the resources provided by the community.

In the modern health system, hospitalization, because of rising cost, is going to be increasingly devoted only to acute, short-term patients. Therefore, the trend for home care worldwide is to enlarge its range of interventions to encompass clinical cases that only a few years ago could have been considered necessitating intensive care in a high-technological hospital unit. The length of hospitalization is also shrinking in some cases to less than half of what it used to be, for comparable clinical conditions, only 2 or 3 years ago. As a consequence, home care nursing is experiencing, in many countries, a dramatic shift of philosophy and activity: from mostly a human, social-health service to a high-technological, medical one. *Hospital at home* is a relatively new term but is already popular within medical language; however, this concept was unthinkable only a few years ago. This new way to manage even critical clinical cases, providing technology and professional support but keeping the patient at home, has already had a great impact on the professional culture. Indeed, this trend is an export of medical culture and high technology from hospital to home caring: a risky trend for those who believe that technology and intensive medical cure do not necessarily mean better quality of care.

Hospital at home may also mean different skills and a different philosophy of approach for nursing at home (client's environment). It also may result in no differences from nursing in hospital, the domain of high technology, medical culture, and clinical skills.

Thus, increasing technology and making the patient's home more hospital-like may end in an extension of the hospital-medical culture, and may overshadow the home care nursing culture. This is a threat and challenge for nursing: a threat because medicine and technology are powerful and often overwhelm any other alternative in Western cultures; and also a challenge because nursing is different in many ways. There is an added value for the patient cared for by a nurse, for the family, and for the entire culture—and the ways our society deals with health, well-being, sufferance, and death.

CONCLUSION

The uniqueness of home care nursing is not only in taking care of the patient at home but also in making more therapeutic the patient's own environment. The uniqueness of nursing at home is in making possible a culture of health and well-being in the patient's home. Through education and stimulation, using communication technique and carefully monitoring attitudes and behaviors, a nurse can activate patient and family resources to achieve the best results. Thus, the nurse serves as a catalyst of the patient's or family's own healing process, and an activator of potentiality, leading toward autonomy and independence, even if the only possible result is the person's death. Therefore, a nurse as a health professional has to be able to perform a reliable assessment and achieve a good understanding of the patient's alterations and potentialities, considering also family dynamics and coping processes. Moreover, a nurse must be able to stimulate, activate, and educate to make the patient's environment therapeutic. A nurse-catalyst is, therefore, an activator of potentiality when that exists but also a direct and effective provider of care when no one else but the nurse can be useful.

What makes the nurse a unique professional for the patient at home? It is the culture of nursing care, in which the person's well-being, not the disease, is the phenomenon of concern. Thanks to that, a nurse is always mindful of freeing the patient from dependence on the caregiver. Providing knowledge, tools, and motivation, the nurse can lead patients and families to make better use of their resources and teach them how to care for and heal themselves.

REFERENCES

Cronin, G., & Harrison, B. (1988). Importance of nurse caring behaviors as perceived by patients after myocardial infarction. *Heart & Lung, 17,* 374–380.

Heller, B. R., Bausell, R. B., & Ninos, M. (1994). Nurses' perception of rehabilitation potential of institutionalized aged. *Journal of Gerontological Nursing, 10,* 22–26.

Lindgren, T., & Linton, D. A. (1991). Problems of nursing home residents: Nurse and resident perceptions. *Applied Nursing Research, 4,* 113–121.

Rieman, D. J. (1986). Noncaring and caring in the clinical setting: Patients' descriptions. *Topics in Clinical Nursing, 8,* 30–36.

Solomon, K. (1982). Social antecedents of learned helplessness in the health care setting. *The Gerontologist, 22,* 282–287.

Trojan, L., & Lange, O. (1993). Developing trusting, caring relationships: Home care nurses and elderly clients. *Journal of Advanced Nursing, 18,* 1903–1910.

CHAPTER 2

Home Health Care Worldwide: An Introduction to Global Issues

Doris M. Modly

INTRODUCTION

Home care, including home-based nursing care, has become a much discussed topic in health care planning and provider circles in the United States as well as worldwide. The interest is spurred not only by rising health care costs, but also by health care consumers' increasing dissatisfaction with the depersonalization of the highly technical and instrumental modern health care in institutional settings. People generally like to be in their own homes in familiar surroundings when ill, and they also recover best at home. This chapter provides an overview of universally experienced problems and issues facing health care systems regarding home-based health care including home nursing. Selected approaches to meeting the needs of specific client cohorts in several countries are presented.

Before home health care in different countries is described, however, home care and, specifically, home nursing must be defined. Jamieson (1991) defines "home care" on the basis of the policies and practices of home care services for older people in Europe. She includes technical nursing, personal care, and homemaking services in the definition, but warns that "in a cross-national survey of home care services the concept would not mean the same thing in all countries" (p. 9). In this chapter, home care refers to home health care as well as to social care in general because it is often difficult to separate the two. A delineation of the two types of services is often based on the sources and amount of financing available. In most countries, financing of the two may be separate, and this can lead to a confusing lack of coordination of services.

HOME CARE STRUCTURES

At a recent home care and hospice conference in Hungary, Karpati (1994) spoke of the challenge in the provision of comprehensive home-based health care. In her thought-provoking and eloquent presentation, Karpati pointed to the need to develop an infrastructure for home-based health care to ensure appropriate development and financing of services provided in the client's home. As an example, she discussed such an infrastructure currently being developed in Hungary. Three service models have been introduced and made available to the public: (a) a government operated and financed model; (b) the so-called privately operated model, which is partly financed by governmental sources and partly by private client sources; and (c) the model operated by private organizations and funded by foundations and charitable organizations as well as government grants. The role of professional nurses in these models is currently being discussed, and nurses are being prepared for the evolving roles of the home care nurse. Karpati (1994) suggested four structural prerequisites to the development of an effective home health care system: (a) the position of home care services in the total health and welfare system of the country, (b) financing of home-based health care, (c) the formulation of standards of care, and (d) planning and development of competent manpower (p. 30).

Karpati (1994) concluded her discussion with a paraphrased saying by Seneca, who suggested that one should first determine what needs to be healed (or changed) and only then should one search for the way to do it (Seneca, n.d.). Considering both points made by Seneca, we need to be clear about what the needs are that must be met, the issues that must be faced, and the problems to be solved. Only then can we search for solutions that respond to the needs within the context of each particular country's reality. The aim of this book is to provide readers an opportunity to learn from one another not only how to provide effective home- and community-based health care, but also to learn what the needs are that cannot be dealt with in various countries because of the lack of material and human resources.

HOME CARE FOR THE ELDERLY

Globally, two groups of clients are in serious need for changes in present systems. These are the elderly and human immunodeficiency virus (HIV)/AIDS-infected individuals. In most cultures, the elderly have traditionally been cared for by their own families. In most countries families are still willing to care for their elders, but families need support to continue in this role (Steel & Gezary, 1994). Further, in countries where the traditional extended family is breaking up because of urbanization or population migrations as country borders are redefined, the cultural norm of care for the elderly within the family and their own home is no longer a feasible solution. In countries of the developed industrial North as well as in the countries of the developing South, the migration of younger families to the cities, or from one city to another in search of employment, contributes to the dissolution of the traditional extended family. The elderly who do not find a place in the industrialized cities are thus left without caregivers. Moreover, as longer life expectancy is achieved for the aging population, the quality of their life deteriorates and becomes a concern.

Efforts to deal with the needs of the elderly are emerging in similar patterns in different parts of the world. Research in the North, or the developed countries, indicates that home care by professional caregivers, specifically nurses, is effective in maintaining wellness in the elderly. For example, a study conducted in Denmark (Hendrikson, Lund, & Stromgard, 1994) found that elders who received wellness visits by nurses in their own homes at least once every 3 months had significantly fewer emergency calls and hospitalizations than elders in the control group.

In Sweden, the concept of the "service house" or sheltered home is a humane alternative to the depersonalization of institutional care, or at the other extreme, the difficulties encountered by the elderly when living alone in their own home. The service house expresses the concept and care of the community for its elders. In Sweden, it is taken for granted that older people have made important contributions to society, and in their later years they deserve a good life and the best that can be offered (Asplund & Bonita, 1994).

African member states of the World Health Organization are also looking for ways to pay special attention to the needs of the elderly within communities to improve the quality of the years that have been added to their life. These new strategies include involvement in community activities through use of their skills, economic independence, and the maintenance of physical fitness (Mihindou-Ngoma, 1994).

Community- and home-based care for elderly psychiatric/mental health patients has been provided in European countries for some time. In Great Britain, Paykel, Mangen, Griffith, and Burns (1982) implemented a controlled trial of routine psychiatric outpatient care and supportive home visiting by psychiatric nurses and discovered that individuals visited by nurses had fewer contacts with psychiatrists, more discharges from care, and only a small increase in general practitioner visits. In The Netherlands, Kerkstra, Castelein, and Philipsen (1991) determined that nurses actively taught self-care skills to older adults during preventive home visits. McDougal (1995) found that 101 older adults discharged from acute care psychiatric hospitals in the United States were able to return home to the community if there was a psychiatric nurse available to make home visits for skilled nursing and supportive psychotherapy. The investigators found that one third of these elderly having combined diagnoses of depression and substance abuse were at increased risk for suicide, and those who had no home visits made more suicide attempts than those visited by psychiatric home visiting nurses. Domiciliary care or nursing care in the home after an acute illness is more effective in restoring the elder's function than a prolonged hospital stay. Research conducted by Currie et al. (1980) demonstrated a faster recovery rate of elders at home than in hospitals. This points to the need to develop domiciliary care for elders both to maintain their level of functioning and to recover from episodes of acute illness. How this will be achieved depends on the context, the country, and its resources as well as the attitude of the community toward the elderly that prevails in a particular society. Prevailing attitudes of health care workers may need to change to facilitate this reorientation to home-based care for elders. Gokhale and Dave (1994) in an article that appeared in a World Health Organization (WHO) publication, *World Health,* raised a fundamental question: How do the elderly, in their own cultural context, view aging, and, therefore, what do they expect from the years that "have been added" to the life of the elderly? Attempts must be made to plan health care for elders in each country in such a way as to be congruent with the cultural values of the society and fit the society where the elder presently lives. In this age of global migrations, however, this is a major issue, particularly when migrations are in the direction of the industrialized, depersonalized countries and away from agricultural countries with close family ties.

HOME CARE AND HIV/AIDS PATIENTS

A second group of clients who are in need of home care and whose problems need "healing" is HIV/AIDS infected individuals. Whatever the effectiveness of efforts to prevent HIV infections, the number of persons becoming ill with AIDS will only increase over the coming years. Because of the chronic nature of the illness, continuity of services between the acute and the chronic phases needs to be assured. Continuity between care provided in the acute care setting and in the home is critical. Communication between caregivers in different care settings is a recurrent topic in home care conferences as well as in the home care literature. There are many reasons why HIV/AIDS patients are better cared for if the patient's own home is the place where most care is given. These reasons include greater flexibility of care, more nurturance, and the proximity of family and friends. In home-based care, there are also opportunities for family members and other caregivers to learn about caring for the patient and to understand the disease. There is less expense for the family and more opportunities for the whole family to carry out their activities with minimal interruption. Anderson and Kaleeba (1994) cite two examples of creative solutions in home care for HIV/AIDS patients. One is the Uganda AIDS Support Organization, TASO, which provides socialization, counseling, medical care, and some income-generating activities for their clients. If the client is too ill, a home care nurse visits and provides care.

Situations of severe poverty and overcrowding that make it impossible for lay or professional caregivers to provide necessary care. For instance, in Zimbabwe or in overcrowded apartments in industrial cities, care units are built where patient and family share a small room and the family provides care for the patient. If the family cannot provide care, a sero-positive individual is trained to give comfort and care for common ailments and needs (Anderson & Kaleeba, 1994). Such partnerships between family and community are essential for future care of the increasing number of AIDS patients globally.

The role of community-based care is emphasized by Anderson (1994), a nurse scientist associated with WHO's Global Program on AIDS. She states that the characteristics of communities lend themselves to coping with the multiple and complex aspects of the AIDS epidemic. Conversely, however, communities need help in overcoming the fear and stigma associated with the disease, thereby bridging the geographical distances between patients and sources of help in confronting the danger of both HIV infection and tuberculosis.

In a report of a study conducted in Rotterdam, The Netherlands, Moons, Kerkstra, and Biewenga (1994) concluded that specialized home care provided by specially trained nurses is effective from the patient's perspective as well as from the perspective of formal and informal caregivers. They found issues emerging around communication and coordination of caregivers and recommended considering these issues more carefully in the future.

Many of the needs of the chronically ill and disabled are similar to those of the elderly and HIV/AIDS patients. The chronically ill, whether young or old, all experience limitation in their activities of daily living. Quality of life questions have to be addressed in addition to needs for medical and nursing care. In Hungary, to overcome the problem of fragmented care, physical and occupational therapists collaborated with home care nurses and family physicians to form home care teams to organize care for elderly patients discharged from hospitals (Karpati, 1994).

HIGH-TECH AND HOME CARE

"High-tech" health care has greatly affected the nature of home care in countries where high-tech medicine is practiced. It affects clients of all ages from the prematurely born to the disabled and ill elderly. User-friendly procedures and high-tech devices are easing self-care as well as care provided by auxiliary helpers. Advances in telecommunication and information management have increased efficiency and access to needed information for caregivers in the privacy of their homes and group support for both patients and caregivers when they need it. Computer-linked support groups of AIDS patients and spouses of post–open heart surgery patients are based on research by Brennan, Moore, and Smyth (1995). The availability of high-tech equipment in the home, however, requires professional home care services for the elderly and chronically impaired persons. This leads to the necessity to educate auxiliary and family caregivers to provide the needed care when the professional caregiver, the home nurse, is not present.

CONTINUING EDUCATION

Continuing education is needed for caregivers, from the family care-giver to the professional specialist, the high-tech expert, or the clinical nurse specialist. All need access to information and training in the special requirements of providing effective, quality care in the home. The concepts of primary, secondary, and tertiary prevention as well as primary; secondary; and, in some instances, tertiary care nursing have to be addressed in educational programs for nurses who will work in home care. Nurses in England and Wales expressed the need for team work and working along with other community health professionals (Atkin, Hirst, Lunt, & Parker, 1994). In the United States, nurses are already being reeducated to a home care orientation in the "retooling" workshops offered to institutionally based nurses who seek to work in the home. Even in basic nursing school curricula, there is greater emphasis on clinical judgment and decision-making skills, interpersonal relationships with family members, and team work. Educational preparation of professional or lay caregivers in the high-tech but home-based setting must ensure technical competence and accountability of caregivers, and a caring attitude expressed in interpersonal skills.

ECONOMICS AND HOME CARE

Issues of cost containment most often trigger the search for effective home care organizational structures. The worldwide need to regulate health care costs is leading to major health care reforms in many countries of the world. Home-based health care has been demonstrated to be cost-effective, and to reduce bills in both operating and capital expenditures for health care. According to Sorochan and Beattie (1994), however, home care is more cost-effective if it is accompanied by a corresponding reduction in hospital and other institutional beds. Targeting of the population most suited for home-based care is also critical to ensure that an appropriate match is maintained between the nature of the care needed by the client and the caregiver's ability to provide that care.

In countries where major social, political, and economic reforms are in progress, how home health care will be structured and financed is a pressing question that will eventually determine the cost-effectiveness of home-based health care (Karpati, 1994). For home care to be effectively structured, the prerequisites for an effective home care system suggested by Karpati must be met: (a) the position of home care, (b) financing of home care, (c) standards of care, and (d) human resource development.

Based on this brief review of the needs and some attempts at solutions, it must be concluded that even though there are global commonalities in health care needs and problems, solutions also have global commonalities; however, there cannot be one single model of home care. Home-based health care will have to be differently structured in different parts of the world, and the preparation and competence of home nursing care providers must be suited to the specific tasks of each country's total system, structure, and resources.

REFERENCES

Anderson, S. (1994). Community responses to AIDS. *International Nursing Review, 41,* 57–60.

Anderson, S., & Kaleeba, N. (1994). The challenge in AIDS home care. *World Health, 47*(4), 20–23.

Asplund, B., & Bonita, R. (1994). Sweden's Service House concept. *World Health, 47,* 28–29.

Atkin, K., Hirst, M., Lunt, N., & Parker, G. (1994). The role and self-perceived training needs of nurses employed in general practice. *Journal of Advanced Nursing, 20,* 46–52.

Blazer, D. G. (1990). Epidemiology of psychiatric disorders and cognitive problems in the elderly. In R. Michels (Ed.), *Psychiatry* (pp. 1–12). Philadelphia: Lippincott.

Brennan, P., Moore, S., & Smyth, K. (1995). The effects of a special computer network on caregivers of persons with Alzheimer's disease. *Nursing Research, 44,* 166–172.

Currie, C. T., Burley, L. E., Doull, C., Ravetz, C., Smith, G. R., & Williamson, J. (1980). A scheme of augmented home care for acutely ill elderly: Report on pilot study. *Age & Aging, 9,* 173–180.

Gokhale, S. D., & Dave, C. (1994). Adding life to years. *World Health, 47,* 23–25.

Hendriksen, C., Lund, E., & Stromgard, E. (1994). Consequences of assessment and intervention among elderly people: A three year randomized control trial. *British Medical Journal, 298,* 1522.

Jamieson, A. (1991). Homecare in Europe: Background and aims. In A. Jamieson (Ed.), *Home care for older people in Europe.* Oxford: Oxford Medical Press.

Karpati, Z. (1994). Az otthoni apolas mint az alapellatas uj eleme. In Otthoni Apolas es Hospice Szolgalat, E. Krasznai (Ed.), Komarom, Hungary: Orszagos Egeszsegbiztositasi Onkormanyzat.

Kerkstra, A., Castelein, E., & Philipsen, J. (1991). Preventative home visits to elderly people by community nurses in the Netherlands. *Journal of Advanced Nursing, 16,* 631–637.

McDougal, G. (1995). Existential psychotherapy with older adults. *Journal of the American Psychiatric Nurses Association, 1,* 16–21.

Mihindou-Ngoma, P. (1994). Care of the elderly: A community health objective. *World Health, 47,* 30–31.

Moons, M., Kerkstra, A., & Biewenga, T. (1994). Specialized home care for patients with AIDS: An experiment in Rottterdam, The Netherlands. *Journal of Advanced Nursing, 19,* 1132–1140.

Paykel, E. S., Shangen, J. H., Burns, T. P., & Ativa, L. (1982). Community psychiatric nursing for neurotic patients: A controlled trial. *British Journal of Psychiatry, 140,* 573–581.

Ratna, L. (1982). Crisis intervention in psychogeriatrics: A two-year follow-up study. *British Journal of Psychiatry, 141,* 296–301.

Sorochan, M., & Beattie, B. L. (1994). Does home care save money? *World Health, 47*(4), 18–19.

Steel, K., & Gezary, H. (1994). Home care in an aging world. *World Health, 47*(4), 3.

CHAPTER 3

Establishing Home Care Services for Children Worldwide

Ida M. Martinson

Caring for an ill child at home is not unusual for families. Indeed, families have been caring for children by themselves for centuries. However, changes in diseases and medical technology, and economic and social trends have changed home care.

NEED FOR CHILDREN'S HOME CARE SERVICES IN A CHANGED ENVIRONMENT

First consider the changes in diseases. In developed countries, during the first half of this century childhood illnesses were mainly acute infectious diseases with a time-limited, usually brief course of illness and then, in many cases, death. In most countries, once deaths from infections and communicable diseases decreased, the disease that was the leading cause of death for children became cancer. (In some countries, pediatric AIDS is now one of the leading causes of death for children.) In developing countries, today, acute infectious diseases continue to take children's lives. However, chronic childhood illnesses are now estimated to affect between 10% and 20% of all children. For example, asthma affects 1 out of 10; diabetes, 1 out of 600; and epilepsy, 1 out of 1,000. Of chronically ill children, 1 out of 6 have a severe chronic illness.

Many children with severe chronic diseases are dependent on sophisticated technology to sustain life, whereas others demand a great deal of caregiving including monitoring, administering treatments, record keeping, and transporting. With the dramatic changes in technology, including the miniaturization of equipment, such as the oxygen tanks, and the portability of equipment, such as in wheelchairs, parents now are assuming major responsibility for care that before only licensed health care professionals would do in the hospital.

It is estimated that in the United States, between 10,000 and 68,000 children are receiving technological care in the home (1987). The Office of Technology Assessment has identified four types of technology-dependent children.

1. Dependent at least part of the day on mechanical ventilators (up to 2,000 in the United States)
2. Dependent on intravenous administration of nutritional substances or drugs (close to 9,000)
3. Dependent daily on device-based respiratory or nutritional support (about 6,000)
4. Dependent on other medical devices that compensate for vital body function, requiring daily or nearly daily nursing care, such as apnea monitoring, renal dialysis (6,000), or other care (up to 30,000)

Technology-dependent children represent a population with unique needs; these children and their families make unique resource demands on society. The parents of these children become professionals for their child, but they need home health care services.

Economic trends include the dramatic increase in hospital costs and equipment. As a result, electronic monitoring, continuous oxygen administration, mechanical ventilation, hyperalimentation, intravenous drug therapy, and peritoneal dialysis are now all being done in the home. Nurses play a pivotal role in these areas, but payment must be made for professional nursing services.

Finally, social trends include the movement toward deinstitutionalization, the increasing number of women in the work force, changes in family structure, and the growing consumer involvement. Deinstitution-alization is related to the concepts of normalization and mainstreaming. Hospital environments are seen as abnormal and strange. In fact, today increased attention is being given to keeping hospitalization for a child to a minimum and trying to keep family life as normal as possible.

The new environment for home care can be illustrated by the variety of situations in one community in South Korea. Winju is a community of 180,000 people about 2½ hours by bus northeast of Seoul. The major crops of Winju are potatoes and corn. This site serves as a 2-week rotation for students from Winju's 2-year School of Nursing and as a 3-week rotation for senior students from Yangsei University. The author was able to visit Winju recently and make a well-baby visit to a country home. The baby was a 1-month-old girl being cared for by her grand-mother. The mother was working and wanted to work. The young baby will not be able to remain with the grandmother too much longer, how-ever, because the grandmother has too much farm work to do.

A rehabilitation center was also visited. This center cares for 20 post–high school, handicapped young adults. They are bused in the morning from their homes and do projects for which they are paid. Eight girls and 12 boys, some mentally retarded and some physically handicapped, with either cerebral palsy or spinal cord injuries were there.

The next visit was to the fifth floor of an apartment building where a 9-year-old boy lived who needed a kidney transplant. At age 5, he was not treated properly for nephrosis, and had a seizure that left him retarded and unable to speak. The mother's kidney was not a match, and no other family member wanted to donate a kidney to the child because of the mental retardation. It is difficult to get organs for donation because of cultural and religious bias against donation of organs. They do not want to mutilate the body even after death.

A visit to a 9-year-old boy with erythema bodusa was also made. All his toes and fingers were missing. The child had skinny legs and arms. Dressings had to be changed 3 times a week, and each dressing change took 1½ hours. We stayed through the first dressing change. The family paid 20,000 won (approximately $20 U.S.) for a nurse to come to do the dressing changes. The money covered transportation costs plus some of the supplies; however, the hospital was supporting the staff members who went to the home to change dressings. At the present time, insur-ance does not cover home care.

ISSUES IN HOME CARE SERVICES FOR CHILDREN

The following questions must be addressed in establishing home care services for children anywhere in the world:

1. *Child- and family-centered programming.* It is crucial to find out what the child and family need, not what is reimbursable. Private funding can help you find out what is truly needed by the family. If you cover only what is reimbursable, chances are that the services will be inadequate, and your program will not work.

2. *Coordination and integration of services.* What is presently available must be identified, and must be used and coordinated.

3. *Community-based staffing.* Nurses should be hired as a "substitute family member"; home health aides and homemakers who live in the community can provide services for families who have a sick or dying child.

4. *Prevention/recovery focus.* The goal is always prevention and recovery. For the dying child, we must ask: How can we prevent a bed sore? How can we prevent pain? What can we do to help the siblings recover from the experience of a dying child?

5. *Early intervention.* It is crucial to provide assistance before problems get worse.

6. *Management of chronic illness/disability.* It is important to ascertain what is needed to maintain or improve the mental and emotional status of the person or the family. A mother called the author about her severely mentally retarded child; after a home visit, the public health nurse who had responsibility for the area was called. She admitted that she knew of the child, but she had not made a single home visit. We need to take a long-term approach—the people in my area are my responsibility.

7. *Delayed or reduced institutionalization.* Nurses can make a profound difference in this area. For example, while being active in helping families care for their dying child at home, the fact that a nurse was on call to the family 24 hours a day and had made arrangements for the child to be admitted to the hospital if needed resulted in a dramatic decrease in rehospitalization.

8. *Case-mix openness.* It is hoped that there can be one organized pediatric home care service and not a special service for childhood

cancer, another one for heart problems, and still another for technology-dependent children. The pediatric home care services should be available for all children in a particular geographic area. Children with cancer have been managed from more than 500 miles away from their home, but there has always been a local nurse who lived close to the family. There is a need to develop nurse-to-nurse consultants.

9. *Fee flexibility.* Payment depends on the type of health care services that the country provides. In the United States, it is necessary to have private funding as well as insurance and government funding to meet the family and child's needs.

PEDIATRIC HOME HOSPICE CARE

When the needs of children worldwide for home care are considered, it must be recognized that nothing would have a greater impact on the quality of life of children than the pediatric home/hospice care. Four out of five children in the world are in developing countries. Therefore, four out of five children with cancer are in the developing world. It is estimated that there are 166,000 children with cancer in the developing world and 34,000 in the developed world.

Nurses must play a key role in developing home care and especially pediatric services that will include services for the dying child. The knowledge needed to do this is already available. The examples presented here from the author's work with dying children can be useful for the development of home hospice care and for other pediatric home care services. The first step is to define what services you will provide and for what reasons. The work began with two questions: Is it feasible for a child dying of cancer to be cared for in the home? Is home care for the dying child and family desirable? The answers to those two questions were not known, so a case study approach was used. Each child referred to this work was managed at home using all the resources necessary. Detailed records, including the time spent on the telephone with the family, what the conversations were about, details of the home visits, and the use of other health care personnel, such as a physician, other nurses, or home health care help, were kept. Reimbursement was pursued whenever possible.

In 1972, home care was provided for Eric, a 10-year-old boy dying of leukemia whose cancer cells had metastasized to his brain. He was becoming increasingly paralyzed. His parents did not know it was possible to care for a child at home, and it was not known if it was feasible or desirable because up to that time most of the author's clinical work had been in the hospital. It was necessary to be on call 24 hours a day, 7 days a week while maintaining the positions of professor and director of nursing research at the University of Minnesota. This experience was life changing. Emmy, the mother of Eric, wrote the following:

> I had never seen anyone die nor had I ever experienced the loss of someone I dearly loved. It was extremely important to me to have been with Eric during the actual transition from life to death, to really know firsthand that it went smoothly for him. The dreaded fear, death, was not ugly as I had thought it would be—Eric was at peace. We, too, had a feeling of peace. Eric's problems were over and we did not have to bear the guilt of not having done all we could for our son. To bear his loss was in itself a great enough burden (E. Vulenkamp, personal communication, 1972).

Several colleagues at the School of Nursing cared for eight more children during a 2-year period. Finally, with major research funding from the National Cancer Institute, a program was set up that provided families who had a dying child with home care services in their home. A geographic area of more than 500 miles was covered. The telephone became a vital link, not only with the family but with the nurse recruited from the family's home community. Because the research funding was limited to 4 years, efforts began almost immediately to incorporate home care services in the major hospitals in the Minneapolis–St. Paul area. The stimulus for the development of home care services at Children's Hospital in Minneapolis and the University of Minnesota were generated through this program.

The author learned from the experience to "keep at it." There are many obstacles, but there is always a way around the various obstacles in providing care (e.g., obtaining sufficient pain medications). Initially, while preparing to provide care for a family, pain medication was one of the first concerns. At that time, the physicians thought that the concerns about children's pain and children's pain medicine were being exaggerated. However, it is now known that most children do have pain. For example, a panic telephone call was received regarding a child's pain resulting from cancer; the physician was quickly reached, and meperidine hydrochloride (Demerol) was ordered, with the hospital providing syringes and needles. The father was taught to give the pain injections. At that point, the author decided that preparation would always be made for managing children's pain in the future.

Two points must be remembered about children with pain. First, because of drug education in the schools, children may be afraid they will become addicted or immune to the effectiveness of the drug. Second, they are afraid they will need to be hospitalized to have pain control. This second myth is frequently believed by nurses and physicians as well as children and family members. The Seattle Pain Clinic for adults suggested trying methadone for a child who was referred to home care while in the hospital and had suffered pain while in the hospital. Methadone was used for many of the children, and the drug was found to be effective. Today, the WHO ladder of pain control is basically the same for children and adults in the type of drugs used. Oral medications can generally be used if an indwelling line has not been inserted. Morphine is the drug of choice. With morphine and other drugs for pain management that need to be given around the clock, constipation quickly becomes a problem. It is important to have the child free of pain to enjoy the last days of life.

Italy has played an important role in the development of a new WHO document on pediatric pain management for children with cancer. A few years ago, Livia Benini died from cancer at home and in pain. Her mother, Franca Benini, was determined to change the situation for other children. Because of her efforts, 25 nurses from around the world were at Castle of Gargonaza in June 1993, where a manual on pain management for children was written. Its amazing how children can respond in their home environment. Bedridden children will frequently even be able to go for tractor rides at home!

The author has had some involvement in the establishment of home care services for children in the United States; Greece; Taiwan, Republic of China; South Korea; China; and other countries. Lessons can be learned from each of these countries in developing home care for dying children.

Taiwan

In Taiwan, after completing a study of the impact of childhood cancer on families in Taiwan, a Childhood Cancer Foundation was developed.

This organization raises funds for the treatment of childhood cancer. The death rate decreased by 33% during a 10-year period. Several nurses are now involved in helping Chinese families care for their child dying from cancer at home. There are plans to develop a more systematic program of hospices in Taiwan. Pain control has also improved dramatically there.

China

In China, there have been two studies completed, one on the impacts of childhood cancer on families and a second on caring for chronically ill children in the home. However, more services are greatly needed for children at home. Presently, children being treated for cancer basically live in the hospital until there are no more funds; then they go home and die without pediatric hospice services. A tremendous difference could be made in the lives of these families if nurses would develop hospice services for the families. Symptom management would be like a miracle to these families and, indeed, for families anywhere who care for their child that is dying. Professor Ma in the School of Nursing in Tianjin, China, has been caring for dying children at home, and the author has personally supported this project for 2 years by providing funds for medications and treatments in the home.

South Korea

In South Korea, hospice has been in existence for some time, and expansion to include children can be easily done. A special project under the direction of Dr. Susie Kim at Ewha Women's University has been established with private funds. A project was completed in South Korea in 1990 that prepared a cadre of nurses, both master's and doctorally prepared, clinicians, and educators/researchers in the area of childhood cancer.

Japan

Home care generally needs to be developed in Japan, especially home services, such as hospice. Hospices exist in Japan, but little home care is provided. However, Japan has the necessary supports for the development of more pediatric services in the home. A few changes would need to be made, but the resources are there. The dominance of physicians is a problem for nursing; in fact, it is only recently that baccalaureate education for nurses has been seen as important for Japanese society. Now there is a surge in baccalaureate education for nurses in Japan.

England

The community nursing organization that England has is to be envied; nursing services are available for both families and children. For example, the children's hospital has a core of nurses who serve the London area, divided into districts. These nurses provide the professional services for families who have a child with cancer, from the time of diagnosis to full recovery, or to death. Bereavement care is also given to the family.

Greece

While at the University of Athens a few years ago, the author participated in a year-long educational program for social workers and nurses to prepare them for the development of pediatric hospice care throughout Greece.

United States

In a recent survey of the more than 2,000 hospices in the United States, 90% said they were willing to provide hospice services for children. The available services have increased tremendously. Special consideration needs to be given to childhood developmental, physical, mental, and emotional issues. Symptom control must be adapted to children, and working with the family is crucial. Last year, a pediatric oncologist requested that the author visit a girl who was dying after a battle with leukemia for 8 years. He was concerned that she was isolated, and no one was talking to her about her feelings. The child's physician was contacted, and he also was interested in the child being visited by a hospice nurse. The mother was telephoned; she wanted a nurse to come, but she would not give permission for the nurse to speak with her child. The decision to visit did not change, as now the concern was not only for the child, but the family too. The family's roots were in the Midwest, which was an area with which the nurse was familiar. While speaking about "the area," the mother seemed to relax and even asked the nurse to have a vegetable salad with her. She shared the medical history of her daughter and that three of her older children were coming, including her husband, for this family conference. The discussion progressed in general terms about the impact of the illness on the family. During this time, three friends came to see the adolescent boy, and he sent them to his room to wait. This was a clear sign that he had serious questions. The first concern was when they needed to take their child to the hospital. The hospital had informed them that they would give the child a blood transfusion, which they did not want because they were Jehovah's Witnesses. When the nurse responded that the child might not need to be rehospitalized, that she could die at home, there was a tremendous release of the tension among the family members. The dying process (and what it would entail) was discussed. Alternatives to hospitalization were offered, such as having the nurse and physician come to the home instead of taking the child to the hospital. It was also suggested that the child might die at home without the need for a health care professional visit, but they should keep their nurse and physician informed. The adolescent son who had chosen to remain in the family group rather than go with his friends had specific questions on what death would be like. A parent's manual was sent to the family, and a telephone call was received about 2 weeks later that their daughter had died at home with the family.

RESOURCES TO ASSIST IN THE DEVELOPMENT OF PEDIATRIC HOME/HOSPICE PROGRAMS

One must be committed, involve others, be persistent, and document the trials along the way to the development of pediatric home care services. Two useful manuals are available in English from Children Hospice International (700 Princess St. Lower Level, Alexandria, VA 22314). The first manual is entitled *Home Care for Seriously Ill Children: A Manual for Parents* by Moldow and Martinson. The second is *Children's Hospice/Home Care: An Implementation Manual for Nurses* by Martinson, Martin, Lauer, Birenbaum, and Eng. The first is useful for families to have available in their homes. It begins by describing home care for the dying child including a section on when to use home care. The second chapter is titled, "Can We Provide Home Care for Our Dying Child?" While parents provide excellent care, they need reassurance, and this chapter provides it. The third chapter is titled, "Is It Time to Stop Treatment?" A few physicians are able to answer parents' questions about ceasing cure-oriented treatment when the parents take the initiative and ask. Frequently, the health care team believes the family is not yet ready to hear the bad news. The fourth chapter in the manual discusses the physical care a child might require at home including information on medications and especially pain control, and prevention and control of other problems, such as bleeding, nausea and vomiting, high fever, respiratory distress, seizures, and constipation. The chapter also includes sections on general care, such as nutrition, mouth care, skin care, eye care, information on the physical activity of the child, and a discussion of health care and equipment. Other chapters include emotional concerns that family members may have and discuss payment for home care, the use of community resources, when funeral and autopsy arrangements should be made, what will happen at death, and whether home care is right for a particular family. When home visits are made, this manual frequently is found in the living room available for the family to read.

The second manual provides step-by-step information for nurses on the development and management of pediatric hospice/home care for children. This manual first discusses the participants in hospice/home care including the family and child, physician, the nurse, and other support persons. Then the manual discusses administration of home care services and includes suggested criteria for the home care service coordinator. The roles of the coordinator at time of referral, the interim period, near death, at death, and after death are also described. This section closes with suggested criteria for the primary nurse. The next section includes a nursing model of care, which includes resource coordination, maintenance of family routines and interaction, and the direct care needed. Another section includes sample forms for physician referral, a child assessment guide, and daily contact records, for example, medication recording. The sixth section includes commonly used medications. The seventh section provides selected analgesics and the eighth section a bibliography. This manual was dedicated to an 8-year-old boy in Iowa who told his mother to share with the author, "A kid ought to decide where he wants to die." His request for home care is the imperative for all of us today.

BIBLIOGRAPHY

Chen, Y., Chao, Y., Martinson, I. M., Lai, Y., Kao, B., & Tseng, G. (1991). The impact of childhood cancer on the Chinese family: A ten year follow-up study (35th Anniversary of National Taiwan University's School of Nursing Research Report No. 89-104). (In Chinese with English abstract.)

Chen, Y. C., Martinson, I. M., Chao, Y. M., Lai, Y. M., & Gau B. S. (1994). A comparative study of health care for children with cancer in 1981 and 1991 in Taiwan. *Pediatric Nursing, 20,* 445–449.

Cho, Y., Kim, S., & Martinson, I. M. (1992). The experiences of parents whose child is dying with cancer. *Korean Academic Society of Nursing, 22,* 512–526.

Fleming, J., Challela, M., Eland, J., Hornick, R., Johnson, P., Martinson, I., Nativio, D., Nokes, K., Ridle, I., Stelle, N., Sudela, K., Thomas, R., Turner, Q., Wheeler, B., & Young, A. (1994). Impact on the family of children who are technology dependent and cared for in the home. *Pediatric Nursing, 20,* 379–388.

Kim, S., Yang, S., & Martinson, I. M. (1992). The impact of childhood cancer on the Korean Family. *Korean Academic Society of Nursing, 22,* 636–652.

Martinson, I. M. (1976). *Home care for the dying child: Professional and family perspectives.* New York: Appleton-Century-Crofts.

Martinson, I. M. (1989). The challenge of culturally diverse pediatric clients. In *Pediatric Nursing Forum on the Future: Looking Toward the 21st Century,* Proceedings and Report from an Invitational Conference, May 16–17, 1988, Fairfax, VA.

Martinson, I. M. (1989). Impact of childhood cancer on family care in Taiwan. *Pediatric Nursing, 15,* 636–637.

Martinson, I. M. (1994). Health care: Responsible social priorities. *Word & World, 14,* 79–81.

Martinson, I. M. (1994). Near-death experiences of children. [Commentary]. *Journal of Pediatric Oncology Nursing, 11,* 145.

Martinson, I. M., & Bossert, E. (1994). The psychological status of children with cancer. *Journal of Child and Adolescent Psychiatric and Mental Health Nursing, 7,* 16–23.

Martinson, I. M., Chang, G. Q., & Liang, Y. H. (1993). Chinese families after the death of a child from cancer. *European Journal of Cancer Care, 2,* 169–173.

Martinson, I. M., Chen, Y. C., Liu, B. Y., Lo, L. H., Ou, J. C., Wang, R. H., & Chao, Y. M. (1982). Impact of childhood cancer on the Chinese families. *Medical Science, 4,* 1395–1415.

Martinson, I. M., Kim, S., Yang, S. A., Young, S. C., Jeong, S. L., & Young, H. L.

(1995). Impact of childhood cancer on Korean families. *Journal of Pediatric Oncology Nursing, 12,* 11–17.

Martinson, I. M., & Liang, Y. H. (1992). The reactions of Chinese children who have cancer. *Pediatric Nursing, 18,* 345–349.

Martinson, I. M., & Liu, B. Y. (1988). Three wishes of a child with cancer. *International Nursing Review, 35,* 143–146.

Martinson, I. M., & Liu, B. Y. (1989). Wishes of children with cancer. *Nursing Times, 85,* 65.

Martinson, I. M., McClowry, S. G., Davies, B., & Kulenkamp, E. J. (1994). Changes over time: Family bereavement following childhood cancer. *Palliative Care, 10,* 19–25.

Martinson, I. M., Yin, S. X., & Liang, Y. H. (1993). The impact of childhood cancer on fifty Chinese families. *Journal of Pediatric Oncology Nursing, 10,* 13–18.

Martinson, P. V., & Martinson, I. M. (1988). The religious response of the Chinese family to childhood cancer. *American Asian Review, 6,* 59–92.

Saiki, S., Martinson, I. M., & Inano, M. (1994). Japanese families who have lost children to cancer: Primary study. *Journal of Pediatric Nursing, 9,* 239–250.

Wang, R. H., & Martinson, I. M. (1982). A study of the impact of the child with cancer on siblings in Chinese family. *The NAROC Journal of Nursing, 29,* 81–91.

Yang, S., Kim, S., & Martinson, I. M. (1992). The experience of families of children being treated for cancer: Sharing the pain. *Nursing Science, 4,* 17–29.

CHAPTER 4

Education for Home Care Nurses

Piera Poletti

Quality of services depends largely on the way professionals provide care. Therefore, human resources need to be considered as the cutting edge for the development of services. Even if technology, devices, and instruments are important, the outcomes for patients' health depend mostly on professional skills to diagnose, choose, and carry out treatments and care, evaluate progress, and establish therapeutic relationships with patients and families.

As working in the community, especially in patients' homes, is different from providing care in a formal institution, caregivers' preparation has to be specifically reconsidered. Knowledge developed has to be considered as a starting point for reanalyzing individual and institutional needs. Requirements are, in fact, different from those in the past because of the new health, economic, and social context.

Basic, advanced, and continuing education for the caregivers who cover the different roles is required. The education system has to be considered as a whole, strictly connected to the development of services. Clinical practice in home care services has to become an integral part of curricula to provide people with knowledge, skills, and attitudes necessary to work in the community setting. Moreover, new strategies have to be experimented within the development of educational programs.

The aim of this chapter is to provide the reader with a framework to discuss educational issues for home caregivers. Training needs, educational contents examples, and strategies are illustrated.

The chapter has been written with a global perspective, considering that boundaries among countries are disappearing. In fact, to communicate is easy and exchanges are promoted among people and institutions through different media and conferences, organizational and functional models can easily be learned and applied, and electronic devices allow access to research results worldwide. Even if a particular example does not apply to a specific situation, the skills and knowledge developed from a methodological viewpoint can help professionals, educators, and administrators in every country.

NEW FRONTIERS IN EDUCATION

First of all, it is important to underline that education must be considered instrumental to the service to be offered to the population. As a consequence, it has to be allocated in a specific context, having a clear idea of the present situation, but also of the future one. In fact, the human resource, if well prepared, cannot just manage the services in a cost-effective way, but must also modify them to adapt to emerging necessities and new requirements. Therefore, the principles that education has to assume are the following: (a) future perspective—in the development of programs, not just current skill training needs have to be considered, but people have to be provided with skills enabling them to face the future demands; (b) person centered—to guarantee that the person will develop self-awareness and the ability to deal with the change and the new requirements and will be able to decide what and how to continue to learn; (c) processes focus—only if a person learns how to analyze, elaborate, interpret, find out new ways of knowing and looking for new solutions can one become an autonomous protagonist of the care delivery. If a person will learn by heart a set of notions, which will soon be old, she or he applies them even if new knowledge is available. Knowledge of the processes could offer a better understanding of patients' situations and better interventions; and (d) teach her or him how to learn. Only if a person recognizes his or her learning style and becomes confident with the learning strategies that are complementary can the probability he or she will use them in the future professional life increase. Another important aspect is the knowledge of all the educational and scientific resources a person can refer to. Sometimes, even if resources are available, professionals do not know about their existence, or how to use them. For example, in many Italian hospitals electronic bibliographical indexes are available, but often nurses do not know about them, or they think only physicians can access and can be interested in using them. To be able to adapt different learning styles and attitudes, education programs have to contain multiple instruments and methodologies including the latest technological ones. Cost-benefits can be the guiding criterion in choosing the didactic tools. Much effort has to be paid to monitor the efficacy of the different educational strategies to provide educators, administrators, and professionals with tools from which to choose.

Another important new development in education is the need for a close relationship between basic and continuing education. In the past, people could rely on the background acquired in school; now they must see themselves as trainees throughout their lives. Therefore, basic and continuing education programs can be mutually supportive, sharing parts of the modules and exchanging tools and faculty.

In this chapter, the education components are discussed according to the preceding principles and the recent literature.

TRAINING NEEDS OF HOME CARE NURSES

As education is an instrument, the first step is to outline the purpose of this instrument. The aim of education in the health care services field is to provide professionals with the knowledge, attitudes, and skills required to accomplish the work. Therefore, it has to be defined first which are the nurses' educational needs that will enable them to work in the home care setting. In the last few years, studies have been carried out about this topic, all underlining its importance. Most of the studies published are focused on "continuing education needs." The findings of the "in-service" studies can, however, be useful for developing or updating the curricula of basic nursing education. To analyze education needs, different approaches have been used, as reported in the following description. Contents identified mostly overlap, even if the more recent data show some differences. More changes in the requirements have to be expected in the future years, as patient populations will increase, mostly because of an earlier discharge from the hospital. In many countries, hospitals at home will become a new reality. Therefore, a different service organization will be designed and new skills will be required by the professionals working in patients' homes. A synopsis of the studies reported in the nursing literature about the topic follows to help the reader to develop new studies or include the information provided in new educational programs.

The needs assessment methodology used to develop an instrument to evaluate nurses' skills before employment is described by Spanier and Gordon (1986). They used the job and documents analysis to identify the nurses' responsibilities. A questionnaire was developed and sent to 200 nursing supervisors to collect opinions about the items chosen. Dela Cruz, Jacobs, and Wood (1986) surveyed the administrators of 254 facilities in four southern California counties, asking them in which areas the greatest educational needs of their nursing staff were. The areas identified were the "basics" of home care, Medicare regulations and documentation, physical assessment, client teaching, and psychosocial skills. Respondents did not believe that basic nursing education prepared nurses adequately to enter the home health field. Nurses were also interviewed in the study (42% had a baccalaureate degree). They believed they lacked skills in the following areas: physical assessment, client teaching and health supervision, nursing diagnosis, family dynamics in home health care, and principles of interviewing and counseling. To produce a tool to use in identifying continuing education needs among in-home nurses, Marter, Becker, Walker, and Sands (1988) surveyed both administrators and field nurses and found nonsignificant differences in rating needs by the two types of subjects. Patient assessment in the home, technical aspects of patient care, legalities of home care, psychosocial aspects, and teaching skills were the need areas identified. Mueller, Johnston, and Bopp (1995) addressed the issue asking the following questions: "What are your community's health problems? Where is nursing practice today? Where will nursing be practiced in 5 to 10 years? What are the five most important outcomes of your educational program today? What are the outcomes needed for future practice?" (p. 24). The approach proposed seems to be appropriate because it relies on a future perspective, refers to the population needs, considers the present professionals, but also designs scenarios for the future. Other authors surveyed training needs from an internal, present-based viewpoint. Caie-Lawrence, Peploski, and Curtis (1995) surveyed nurses and defined training needs as those practice areas home care professionals rated, when requested, highest in importance but lowest in competence. When not only field nurses, but also supervisors and administrators filled in the research questionnaire, many areas of competence, not related to the present tasks, were not rated as important because respondents were focused on themselves and their present work perspective. These authors considered tasks as the reference point to analyze the needs. This approach could limit the professional position, where regulations and organizational boundaries often do not allow one to express all the professional potentialities and sometimes fails to satisfy patients' needs. This is why training needs assessments have to start from a broader perspective and consider the potential for people to learn abilities that allow them to gain a wider horizon to be able to adapt to future requirements and propose and introduce changes. In the cited study, the priority needs identified are the following: physical assessment (i.e., abdomen, gastrointestinal, respiratory, and eyes, ears, nose, and throat), malpractice, agency and third-party regulations, body mechanics, nursing diagnoses, and universal precautions. The authors expressed their concerns for the absence of the following areas among the important ones: coordination of services, computer literacy, and substance abuse. Social and personal changes have a serious impact on many groups in the population. Psychological and psychiatric diseases often come along with other needs. Home care nurses can meet patients who have, in addition to other clinical problems, this kind of need. Therefore, it is important that any home care nurse is able to deal with situations like alcoholism, suicidal attitudes, depression, and so on. Wang, Lee, and Mentes (1995) surveyed 27 nurses from three community health agencies about their knowledge and attitude toward suicide and saw the preparation was insufficient. In the conclusion of the study, they recommend including interventions related to suicide prevention in basic and continuing education.

To get insights about the future perspectives, Manuel and Sorensen (1995) conducted a study to determine the hiring trends of nurses and the expectations for their competencies. With a convenience sample of executives from 96 institutions and agencies across Massachusetts, they asked the following: (a) What are the hiring trends for the professional nurse and unlicensed assistive personnel in hospitals and agencies in Massachussets? (b) What are the skill expectations for professional nursing staff? (c) How are baccalaureate nurses used now, and how will they be used in the future? (d) What nursing skills will be necessary for the future? (p. 250). The results show that in a scenario where there is expected to be an increase of unlicensed assistive personnel, the role of nurses is seen as more managerial. As a consequence, the skills more frequently cited by the respondents are (a) assessment, (b) clinical technical skills, and (c) organizational skills (leadership, critical thinking, delegation and supervision, and communication).

BASIC, ADVANCED, AND CONTINUING EDUCATION

Referring to the domain of training needs for home care, described earlier, basic and continuing education programs can be developed. In an international perspective, even if general program contents are the same, the specific content can be different. For example, law and regulations, economics and reimbursement, and organizational procedures are different among countries. Moreover, the time when a specific skill is required to be learned can be different among professionals from different countries and also from different agencies in the same area, according to the characteristics and the demands by the organizations. It is important for faculty, educators, and executives to have a clear idea of the training needs of home care nurses to assess and plan courses and curricula.

Another important issue at the present time refers to which educational objectives have to be pursued in basic and advanced courses. As a consequence of the hiring trends, Manuel and Sorensen (1995) found that more leadership preparation was expected from baccalaureate nurses to have them supervising and managing other professionals. Therefore, if clinically qualified nurses assume this kind of responsibility, other specific managerial roles will be less necessary. Economic restrictions present a different scenario and the complete set has to be rearranged. It is important that population needs are considered central and the services offered are designed to meet the needs in an efficient way. Even if it is difficult to change the previous perspective a positive approach must be undertaken to find the best solutions. Advanced education must include specific roles professionals are expected to assume; therefore, these roles have to be first outlined, according to the future scenario.

Another challenge education has to face, worldwide, is to prepare for dealing with diversity. In many European countries, people from different cultures have to learn to live together. Nursing schools have to prepare nurses to care for people with different backgrounds in ethnicity, language, and culture. They are also expected to work in interdisciplinary teams effectively. Often they are taught how to work with others, but only if they really learn to work together and discover the advantages of doing so will they learn and continue to do so during their professional life. Waite, Harker, and Messerman (1994) emphasized the need to evaluate the effectiveness of diversity training and to teach the communication process, stressing "diversity" background and contents. Carpenter (1995) described a successful experience of "interprofessional education," involving nurses and doctors who changed their reciprocal attitudes after just a 1-day course together. As in the future, many challenges have to be faced together by health professionals. To provide the best care, in different organizational scenarios, there have to be offered many opportunities to share during the basic education to learn to cooperate in practice.

Faculty preparation to manage the change in curricula development and teaching is especially important. In fact, if the faculty background and expertise are not in the new fields, such as home care, their attitudes toward introducing change and its acceptance by students can be difficult. Mueller, Johnston, and Bopp (1995) suggested promoting actions to overcome this problem, such as seminars for faculty on home care clinical issues and new teaching approaches, and summer practice in-services in which they are less comfortable. Faculty are the role models students first meet; it is important they have a positive attitude and enthusiasm toward what they teach to increase students' motivation and interest.

Many institutions are working on curriculum development. A few examples are summarized here from the nursing literature. However, it seems useful to report first Manuel and Sorensen's (1995) recommendations for redesigning curricula. They stressed the necessity to introduce at the beginning of the classes opportunities for students to develop critical thinking and independent decision making; participate in their learning process both individually and as a group; think conceptually and translate concepts into practical problem solving; learn leadership and organizational skills, and clinical skills in speciality areas, such as community, ambulatory settings, and long-term care, to assess and provide care across the continuum; and, most importantly, understand the health care costs and fiscal management, politics/policy development, and ethics. Mueller et al. (1995) added to this list the nursing process as a key element of the curriculum.

Long (1995) reported the core and the main features of the course in home health care nursing included in the curriculum developed at Arizona State University College of Nursing. The experience is a good example of the need and possibility of collaboration between all the subjects involved in the home care professional education, such as the Home Care Advisory Board, the Home Care Nursing Project staff, health care practitioners and administrators in the community, and the College of Nursing faculty, to obtain a relevant educational project. The main course objectives pursued in the program were the following: (a) assess the patient/family for unmet health needs; (b) assess the environment, including socioeconomic status, culture, and physical surroundings, on the delivery of home health care to patients/families; (c) use nursing diagnosis in the development of the care plan; (d) plan health care in the home in relation to other health services or other health providers in the community; (e) implement plans for intervention in collaboration with the patient/family; (f) actively involve the patient/family with health care teaching activities; and (g) evaluate patient/family interventions as related to goals and expected outcomes.

Bunn (1995) described the course initiated at University of Ottawa on community mental health nursing. A previous survey by the same author had showed that only one school was offering the course, even though patients with psychiatric problems were increasing in number. Polmer (1995) reported on a course introduced in students' junior year on childbearing and family.

Scannel (1995) described the role of the home health clinical specialist as "camouflaged" because of many factors, such as restrictive laws; lack of a specific clinical base for home care specialization, which is a broad field; confusion from not having expert nurses, who, if they are the only ones patients get to know, are considered "experts" and as a consequence no need for further abilities is perceived. Another important issue is the "two wings curriculum," which is the advanced program to be administrative or clinical, or both. To explore this point, Bryant and Cloonan (1992) surveyed faculty and home health care personnel about curriculum content. They focused on two different curricula: one clinically focused and one administrative centered. Main content areas of the clinical curriculum included home health concepts, such as reimbursement regulations, documentation and quality assurance, care of the acutely ill, care of the chronically ill, epidemiology, and community health concepts, such as working with groups and family assessment, nursing theory, and teaching learning theory. Research, policy, and geriatrics also were suggested. Essential contents of the administrative curriculum were identified as the following: home health concepts, financial management, management principles, program development, marketing, organizational theory, and epidemiology. In addition, legal issues and computers were indicated.

As the number of professionals in home care services will increase in the next years, it is urgent to provide knowledge of effective programs for in-service and continuing education to help administrators and educators choose contents and strategies. Therefore, projects tested through research methodology are strongly recommended. Few research-based educational projects were described in continuing education. Cronin-Stubbs et al. (1994) reported on a program called "Motivation of Older Adults," attended by nursing home and home health agencies personnel. The use of the program's contents in their nursing care was analyzed using multiple research methodologies. Many similar types of projects need to be promoted with a cross-cultural focus to obtain a wider base of knowledge on the topic.

STRATEGIES AND DIDACTIC METHODOLOGIES

Education strategies and didactic methodologies have to be multiple during basic, advanced, and continuing education. At the present time, in the multimedia and computerized world, all the "distances" have to be overcome. Students and nurses from different areas, states, and cultural backgrounds have to be given the opportunity, if they have the requisites, to attend programs. Therefore, the educational institutions have to provide flexible systems of structured courses, self-learning packages (audio, video, computer software, and compact disks), distance learning, teaching and coaching, even through electronic networks. If students are used to approaching these media from the beginning of their education, it will be easier for them to continue to update throughout the learning period. Even if there are experiences carried out using the new technologies, not many are described in the recent literature. Anderson (1995) reported on the electronic mail use and its efficacy in strengthening students' feedback and support. Hoeksel and Moore (1994) described the use of computers for clinical skills. Hekelman, Niles, and

Brennan (1994) organized a continuing education system for home care nurses. Providing computer skills, they enable people to access scientific literature specific for the field and a consultant available on line.

During basic education, didactic methodologies have to allow students to become autonomous and be able to perform at the level described previously. Student-centered teaching requires the use of participation methodologies. A description of the important ones, along with research results supporting their potentialities and limits, was offered by McCarthy (1995). Group discussions and seminars to promote a deep understanding of learning as well as attitudes; guided design for decision making; and simulation, games, and role plays for the acquisition of interpersonal skills, attitudes, and problem solving are just a few examples of different methods that can be used. Warner, Ford-Gilboe, Laforet-Fliesser, Oson, and Ward-Griffin (1994) developed a research project, in which the aim was to describe teamwork and factors influencing its development. Pairs of students were offered the possibility to share responsibilities during home care clinical training. Even if many students recognized the usefulness of the "peer work," they really only shared moderately. In their conclusion, the authors stated the usefulness of the shared assignment method of clinical instruction, but agreed on the necessity that it be carefully constructed and monitored. Previous readings and class work on teamwork were considered essential.

A survey carried out by Alley, Donckers, and King (1992) indicated that the considered master's programs in home health care nursing were designed to individualize learning experiences for both experienced and novice nurses to maximize learning. However, little is reported about what activities were carried out to individualize the learning experiences. The wish is that more education experiences will be conducted, also using a research approach, and published to share what will be produced worldwide. Professionals in all the countries must be encouraged to write about their experiences.

REFERENCES

Alley, J. M., Donckers, S. W., & King J. C. (1992). Integrating experienced and novice nurses into graduate home health education. *Journal of Nursing Education, 31,* 357–360.

Anderdon, D. G. (1995). Elecronic education. *Nurse Educator, 20*(4), 8–11.

Bryant, S., & Cloonan, P. (1992). Graduate home health education: A survey of home health educators and agency personnel. *Journal of Nursing Education, 31,* 29–32.

Bunn, H. (1995). Preparing nurses for the challenge if the new focus on community mental health nursing. *The Journal of Continuing Education in Nursing, 26,* 55–59.

Caie Lawrence, J., Peploski, J., & Curtis, R. J. (1995). Training needs of home health care nurses. *Home Health Care Nurse, 13*(2), 53–61.

Carpenter, J. (1995). Interprofessional education for medical and nursing students: Evaluation of a programme. *Medical Education, 29,* 265–272.

Cronin-Stubbs, D., Duchene, P., LeSage, J., Dean-Barr, S., DiFilippo, J. M., Kopanke, D., Stehlin, M., & Swanson, B. (1994). Evaluating a geriatric rehabilitation continuing education program for nursing home and home health agency nurses. *Applied Nursing Research, 7,* 91–93.

dela Cruz, F., Jacobs, A., & Wood, M. (1986). The educational needs of home heath nurses. *Home Health Care Nurse, 4*(3), 11–17.

Hekelman, F. P., Niles, S. A., & Brennan, P. F. (1994). Gerontologic home care: A prescription for distance continuing education. *Computers in Nursing, 2,* 106–109.

Hoeksel, R., & Moore, J. F. (1994). Clinical nursing education at a distance: Solving instructor interaction problems. *Journal of Nursing Education, 33,* 178–180.

Long, C. O. (1995). Home health care: The curriculum mandate. *Home Health Care Nurse, 13*(6), 46–50.

Manuel, P., & Sorensen, L. (1995). Changing trends in health care: Implications for baccalaureate education, practice and employment. *Journal of Nursing Education, 34,* 248–253.

Marter, L., Becker, H., & Walker, L. (1988). Home health care nurses and quality care: Identifying the important skills. *Caring, 7*(10), 38–40.

McCarthy, G. (1995). Research on teaching methods in nursing. In D. M. Modly, R. Zanotti, P. Poletti, & J. J. Fitzpatrick (Eds.), *Advancing nursing education worldwide* (pp. 45–58). New York: Springer.

Mueller, A., Johnston, M., & Bopp, A. (1995). Changing associate degree nursing curricula to meet evolving health care delivery system needs. *Nurse Educator, 20*(6), 23–28.

Palmer, N. S. (1995). Moving student clinical experience into primary care settings. *Nurse Educator, 20*(4), 12–14.

Spanier, A., & Gordon, B. (1986). Assessing pre-employment home health care nursing skills. *Caring, 5,* 60–73.

Waite, M. S., Harker, J. O., & Messeerman, L. I. (1994). Interdisciplinary team training and diversity: Problem, concepts and strategies. *Gerontology & Geriatrics Education, 15*(1), 65–82.

Wang, W., Anderson, F. R., & Mentes, J. C. (1995). Home health care nurses' knowledge and attitudes toward suicide. *Home Health Care Nurse, 13*(5), 64–69.

Warner, M., Ford-Gilboe, M., Laforet-Fliesser, Y., Olson, J., & Ward-Griffin, C. (1994). The teamwork project: A collaborative approach to learning to nurse families. *Journal of Nursing Education, 33*, 5–13.

PART II

Home Care Nursing in Specific Countries

CHAPTER 5

Home-Based Care
in Zimbabwe

Auxilia Munodawafa and
Patricia E. McDonald

In Sub-Saharan Africa, people have faced calamities brought about by disease, famine, drought, and civil wars for generations. Yet the extended family and kinship networks that are the backbone of the African social structure have been able to facilitate the management of these catastrophes. The same region is now facing a different dilemma, and one that the extended family network is finding increasingly difficult to contain—that of AIDS.

AIDS was first recognized in Zimbabwe in 1985. However, at that time its significance as a major public health threat was not fully understood. Since then, the incidence of reported AIDS cases has increased dramatically, a trend that is expected to continue throughout the 1990s (Zimunya, 1992). According to the 1994 *Annual AIDS Report,* current estimates indicate that 800,000 to 1,000,000 persons are HIV positive, including up to 40% of antenatal mothers. A recent study by the Ministry of Health and Child Welfare shows that the prevalence of HIV in both antenatal mothers and sexually transmitted disease patients has increased tremendously. Figures obtained from the 1994 annual report, through the Health Information Unit in Zimbabwe, reveal the distribution of HIV infection by age, sex, province, and national level. Moreover, one quarter of AIDS cases are infants, with the peak occurrence in women who are in their 20s and men in their 30s. These persons with HIV require long-term medical care as they develop recurrent opportunistic infections, such as tuberculosis, chronic diarrhea, and other serious health problems.

Many of these individuals need support and care in the home because hospital services are overburdened and ill-equipped to meet their care needs. Additionally, hospital services and other welfare organizations are experiencing increasing difficulty in meeting care needs, because of global recession and the Economic Structural Adjustment Programs (ESAP) (Zimunya, 1992). One of the most significant negative effects of ESAP has been a sharp increase in unemployment, as government departments as well as the private sector trim down their work forces. In addition, reintroduction of hospital medical fees through cost recovery exercise has imposed a strain on the Department of Social Welfare by increased claims in general.

AIMS OF HOME-BASED CARE

AIDS is a chronic disease lasting months or years. A person with AIDS may move several times from home to the hospital and back home again. Much of the care of those with AIDS, however, occurs in the home. The primary aims of home-based care for persons with HIV/AIDS include (a) prevention of problems when possible, (b) management of existing problems, and (c) knowledge of when to seek help. Home care in Zimbabwe also aims to empower health care workers with the information they need to help families gain confidence in their own ability to give safe, compassionate, and effective care to persons with AIDS in their homes. Within many families and communities, meeting the most basic needs, such as food, clothing, and housing, is problematic. Caring for persons with AIDS creates many additional demands on family and community resources. It is not usually expensive equipment or medicines that are needed, but supplies, such as clean water, soap, essential medicines, and other items, commonly found in homes. In addition, caring family members are essential.

Home care involves the provision of holistic care, which includes (a) medical and nursing care, (b) training of caregivers in the home, (c) counseling and psychological support to persons with AIDS and family members, (d) financial and practical support, and (e) referral to other persons of the multidisciplinary team. Holistic home care provides training for family members to cope with the needs of the patient as well as psychosocial, spiritual, practical, financial, and material support for caregivers and dependents. Lastly, it provides the opportunity to plan for the future with respect to orphans and other dependents.

ORGANIZATION OF HOME-BASED CARE PROGRAMS IN ZIMBABWE

A multisectoral approach in planning and implementation of community-based care has been established at central, provincial, district, and institutional levels (National AIDS Control Program [NACP], 1993). The agents involved include the Ministry of Health and Child Welfare, mission hospitals, clinics registered with the Zimbabwe Association of Church-Related Hospitals, private practice, armed services, medical insurance companies, city health departments, and the informal or traditional sector, Zimbabwe National Traditional Healer's Association (ZINATHA), traditional birth attendance, and others (NACP, 1993). Most services are provided through government and city health department in urban areas, and through mission hospitals in rural areas (*Quarterly AIDS Report,* 1994).

Community-based health care pilot projects have been undertaken in several districts throughout the country. National strategies and guidelines have also been established. Community and clinic nurses under the Department of Community Nursing and Mission Services have provided community outreach services as well. Rehabilitation technicians have been trained and deployed in some district hospitals with the intention of providing a link between the community and hospital services. The NACP, which was established in 1987 by the Ministry of Health, is involved in training health workers in AIDS counseling through workshops.

A study aimed to document AIDS programs in Zimbabwe was conducted by the School of Social Work, Harare, Zimbabwe (Zimunya, 1992). In the study, home care teams were found to be composed of the primary health care nurse, minister, enrolled staff nurse, health educator, teacher, occupational therapist, social worker, community health worker, environmental health technician, rehabilitation assistant, Red Cross, community volunteers, or relatives.

One or two teams involved a doctor, whereas in another scheme, the hospital matron led the team. In one or two hospitals, many nurses (up to 21) had been trained in home care, and in these hospitals, nurses made referrals to teams of community volunteers covering various geographic areas. One program was found to use an HIV-positive counselor openly as part of the home care team. A few programs held regular support meetings for the home care team. At the national level, a committee composed of representatives from the Department of Social Welfare, private sector, Ministry of Health and Child Welfare, nongovernmental organizations (NGOs), religious groups, and support groups of people living with HIV/AIDS provides overall support and coordination of community-based care (Ndimande, 1994). This is being achieved primarily through various multidisciplinary programs.

The NACP, which was established by the Ministry of Health, is involved in training health workers in AIDS counseling through workshops. National strategies and guidelines on community-based care have been established. A subcommittee on community-based care has also been established to provide technical support and enhance coordination of home-based care activities (Ndimande, 1994). There are several distinct programs since 1991. However, levels of implementation including quality of service differ from province to province and within districts within the same province.

There are four major established programs in Harare, Bulawayo, Mutare, Kariba, Chegutu, and Esigodini. It was found that urban programs tended to be based within NGOs and AIDS Service Organizations, whereas rural schemes were based in mission and district hospitals and clinics. Most programs were found to be institutional as opposed to community based, taking the form of outreach services from hospitals or clinics. In some programs, referral chains had been established from hospitals, to clinics, then to community volunteers. It must be remembered that these programs are still in their early developmental stages.

The frequency of visits varied widely from teams visiting patients once a month or once a week to Island Hospice, whose staff visits a patient more than once a day in crisis situations. These visits were reported to last from a range of a few minutes to several hours when practical household tasks and nursing care were provided. Services are provided according to identified needs in the community, and according to money and other resources of the service agency. The basic needs for AIDS patients are finance, employment, family support, nursing care, spiritual support, and nutritional guidance (Mbetu, 1992).

Services that were identified as essential for home-based care are as follows: social support, information, financial support, psychological support, spiritual support, dietary requirements, physical care, medical help for persistent diarrhea and loss of weight, skin problems, bed sores, chest pains, tuberculosis, and a variety of other health-related problems. The primary needs for caregivers in the family were established as financial and material assistance, spiritual and emotional support, and relief from the extra workload of washing bed linens and clothing, running the household, and providing nursing care to the person with AIDS.

ZINATHA's Role in Home-Based Care

One of the most unique groups involved in home-based care in Zimbabwe and in Africa is, no doubt, the traditional healer. In Zimbabwe, when someone leaves the hospital and returns home, a traditional practitioner usually becomes the caregiver in many cases. In the current HIV/AIDS epidemic, most of the practitioners will manage opportunistic infections related to AIDS, such as diarrhea, cough, or skin conditions. ZINATHA works in collaboration with national organizations, such as the National Family Planning, the Zimbabwe Community health counselors, political party leaders, and heads of educational and religious institutions in various programs.

ZINATHA is coordinating in the procurement and distribution of condoms for prevention of sexually transmitted diseases. ZINATHA is also involved in community-based peer counseling groups. The group is currently involved in clinical trials, information, education, and communication. A book in Shona on traditional AIDS education has just been released by ZINATHA. Workshops and seminars have been organized for traditional healers on the clinical care of persons with HIV infection, and a disease management guideline for its members is being compiled.

ADVANTAGES OF HOME CARE

Home-based care is often the best way to manage persons with AIDS. The ultimate wish of many HIV sufferers is to be at home with their

families and friends in familiar, nonthreatening, and private surroundings where they can tie up loose ends and say their good-byes. People
who are sick or dying would rather stay at home (and use the extended
family system), particularly when they know they cannot be cured in
the hospital. Ill persons are comforted by being in their own homes and
communities surrounded by family and friends.

Home care can mean that hospitals are less crowded, so that doctors,
nurses, and other hospital staff can give better care to those who need
to be in the hospital. It is usually less expensive for families to care for
someone at home; for example, they do not have to pay hospital bills
and transportation to and from the hospital. If the sick person is at home,
family members find it easier to meet their other obligations than if the
ill member were hospitalized.

FUNDING

Various organizations have their own sources of funding. Some organizations seek funds from national and international sources for specific
program development. Home care services, likewise, have designated
funding for training, staff development, transport, or nursing kits. Other
organizations have sought funds locally to establish benevolent funds
or material assistance for such items as vegetables, milk, clothes, and
blankets. Examples of such programs are Mashambazhou, in Harare,
which rely on both national and international individuals and groups,
and Zororo, which is ministry sponsored (Mabeza, 1992).

In the case of government services based at district hospitals and
clinics, there seems to be no money earmarked for home care beyond
funding programs that are provided by NACP. The AIDS home care
program is usually an integrated program built into existing community
and health care services to minimize expenses. Such programs include,
but are not limited to, maternal and child health, monitoring of tuberculosis, hypertension, persons with other chronic illnesses and disabilities, and immunization programs. Home visits to patients with AIDS
may be made when the team or the community nursing sister is making
other domiciliary calls. Environmental health technicians based in community clinics also make home calls and are, in some cases, visiting
AIDS patients. Inadequate funding is a major problem on many of the

home care programs and has implications for the sustainability of the programs. In particular, funding is needed to provide transportation, basic nursing kits, and material provisions for destitute families. In many cases, increased staffing levels are also needed as well as funding to give bonuses to volunteers.

PROBLEMS

Referral networks are highly variable, with frequent, serious breakdown in communication and cooperation. There is limited material and financial support because of lack of funding. Patients from rural areas where home care schemes are not available are difficult to refer; therefore, follow-up is not possible. In outreach schemes, primarily referral services and basic advice on nutrition and hygiene are provided during the visits rather than actual medication or nursing care. Confidentiality appears to be a major impediment to effective referral for home care as the family has to have the diagnosis explained to them to accept responsibility of caring for a person with AIDS. Transport is a problem for many programs, also limiting the number of patients who can be visited as well as decreasing the service to those far away from the home care's base. This reduces the effectiveness of home care schemes. Finally, there are no established clear lines of responsibility for home care programs and many patients and families are in desperate need of basic supplies, such as food, soap, detergents, and blankets.

CASE STUDY

Family Background

Tamuka, born September 17, 1957, was born in a family of nine children, being the seventh born. His name, in the local language denotes, "The family name can now be carried on." Simply because Tamuka was the first boy after a chain of six girls, he was the apple of everyone's eye, not to mention his father.

Education

Tamuka completed his secondary education and went on to train as a motor mechanic. Soon after the country's independence, he was one of the lucky ones to be sent to Canada to train in the instructor's course in 1982. On his return, he secured a lectureship's position with one of the technical colleges in Zimbabwe. At the time of his death, he was head of the Motor Mechanic Department.

Social History

He was a stable, level-headed person, one who would not be associated with promiscuity. He had had a bad hand in marriage, however. He married and divorced twice before settling with the last wife, who was a medical doctor and had trained in Cuba for 7 years. Six months into this particular marriage, he suffered from herpes zoster. Thereafter, his health was never the same.

History of Illness

Two or so months after the herpes, Tamuka started having attacks of headaches, which would make work impossible and require stronger analgesics each time. He went through all sorts of investigations including computed tomographic scans until almost a year after, when he was diagnosed with cryptococcal meningitis. Tamuka came from a family background full of medical people who included two sisters who were registered nurses, and a wife who was a medical doctor. Cryptococcal meningitis, from experience, was almost always known to be associated with the HIV infection. So one can imagine the shock, panic, and denial that went through this family. Within a month of the diagnosis, he became more ill and required hospital admission every 2 weeks or so with problems ranging from severe headaches to cardiac disorders and fungal infections. He also tested HIV positive at this time.

Home-Based Care

The care within the next 4 months included mostly home care other than several admissions. He basically lived between the ward and home.

Because of his social position in the family, everyone felt they had to take care of him. This, on occasion, caused friction between his wife, who believed she knew what was best for him as a medical doctor; his two registered nurse sisters, who thought that nurses knew the most about health care; and his mother, who knew what was best for him from birth. This discord resulted in the patient not getting the best care he should have had. He had all the pain killers needed from his wife, and the social and psychological support from the rest of his family and parents. The support, though, was haphazardly given because the whole group remained in denial.

Social Impact

Tamuka's illness and eventual death shattered everyone's dreams. Remember, he was the apple of everyone's eye. All dreams by both parents and siblings were built around him. He had a good education, a good job, and was going up the career ladder quickly. All of a sudden, plans had to change. Financially, Tamuka had taken over all family responsibilities because his father had retired. His two twin brothers, who had been born 7 years after him, though already working, had always been considered babies and, hence, never felt the need to be responsible. Therefore, they were not prepared to take on these responsibilities. His frequent admissions, drugs, and investigations took most of his financial resources. Tamuka's admissions became more frequent until he needed 24-hour nursing care, which was obtained from nursing services. Early on the morning of November 21, 1992, he died in the hospital. His death robbed his wife of a husband at the tender age of 33 years, his four children of a father, his parents and the rest of the family of their apple "Tamuka," and the country of a young motor mechanic lecturer, whom the country had invested in not so long before to go to Canada. The cream of the country had been taken by the killer disease AIDS.

CONCLUSION

Transport is essential for home care teams, in particular, transport to the hospital and transport on discharge from the hospital. Also, transport of deceased persons with AIDS is essential. Additionally, clear lines of responsibility are needed for home care rather than home care being integrated with other activities (e.g., maternal and child welfare, immunizations, and so forth). Home care services should attempt to meet basic requirements for the programs to be effective. Referral systems should be established well ahead of service provision, and clear, simple referral forms are needed. Guidelines as to who has what responsibility should be established including the services available. Involvement of home care providers should start while the patient is still in the hospital, beginning with counseling. There is a need to expand and increase access to and provide quality comprehensive community-based care services to all levels of primary health care.

REFERENCES

The care of the HIV patient at home: A self-study module for rural nurses (1994). Unpublished manuscript, Harare, Zimbabwe.

Mabeza, W. N. (1992). *Community-based care, HIV and counseling activities,* Unpublished manuscript, Harare, Zimbabwe.

Mbetu, P. (1992). *Chitungwiza home based care: National AIDS Program.* Unpublished manuscript, Chitungwiza, Zimbabwe.

National Aids Control Program (1994). *National Public Health Laboratory.* Harare, Zimbabwe: Author.

Ndimande, E. (1994). *Report of the community home-based care programs.* Harare, Zimbabwe: National Aids Coordination Programme.

The Population Council (1993). The Second Medium Plan (MTP2), 1994–1998 (Research Series). *Journal of Social Development in Africa, 3,* 8–12.

Quarterly AIDS Report. (1994). Department of Epidemiology and Disease Control, Harare, Zimbabwe.

Zimunya, V. (1992). Documentation of home-based care programs in Zimbabwe, School of Social Work. *Journal of Social Development in Africa, 3,* 10–11.

CHAPTER 6

Home Care in Belgium

Ludo Geys

During the second part of the 20th century, a new trend surfaced in favor of home nursing in Belgium. The first organized services for home nursing were created around the years 1937 to 1938, and centers were established throughout the country, mainly stimulated by the White and Yellow Cross. After the 1950s, home care went through an uninterrupted expansion, which resulted in several legislative decisions—in particular, the Royal Decree of December 27, 1950, which recognized home care as a part of health care policy.

At a time when other kinds of assistance in the home had been developed (especially domestic and geriatric help as well as social services) and when general practitioners were gaining a greater role, people progressively became aware that cooperation would be the first step toward a more comprehensive home care. Home care is defined as "providing for patients, within a coordinated framework, in their homes a range of different services limited in time and scope that enables the beneficiary to remain within their familiar environment in the best possible conditions."

Professional home care involves four professional services: general practitioners, home nursing, domestic and geriatric help, and social services. These are mostly private services not connected with hospitals. Given the fact that these services fulfill an indispensable role in health care as a whole, the national and community legislations (decrees) have subjected home care to an increasing set of regulations.

Most home care patients (approximately 80%) require and receive monodisciplinary help. For the remaining 20%, once the need for care becomes more complex and more than one professional must intervene, a comprehensive provision of care must be organized. This cannot be done without structured communication systems between the different professionals, who are in charge of home care finance. However, stating this is not enough; logical solutions must be developed by cooperating professionals so that clients' needs can be met. Monitoring this care process (such as guaranteeing the quality and permanency of care as well as empathy) is a job preferably left to nursing specialists.

HOW IS HOME CARE ORGANIZED IN BELGIUM?

When one speaks of "care at home," the first person to come to mind is the general practitioner. Yet, of all home care providers, the nurse is the one who does the greatest number of house visits and who is involved in the highest number of illness cases. Consequently, he or she should play a significant role in the care process.

What Are the Existing Services?

Home care organizations were stimulated via the important health benefit funds in Belgium. For instance, the Christian health benefit fund officially supported the White and Yellow Cross when it decided that all of its members would join that organization. This was not accidental. The White and Yellow Cross was developed in 1937 as a Christian-inspired association, and it took the first steps toward organized home nursing. In 1994, the White and Yellow Cross enjoyed a market share of 50% in Belgium; this means that one half of the expenses of the National Institute for Health Insurance, or about 200 million dollars, are paid to the White and Yellow Cross for nursing care provided by its nurses. Home nursing is also provided by independent nurses.

Organization and Structure

The policies and development of an organized service for home nursing are based on the following principles:

- Division of labor
- Continuity of care, each day or several times a day, including on Sundays and holidays
- Provision of all types of care, in particular long-term care for highly dependent patients
- Wide range of nursing activities
- Help for all sick people, wherever they live, without any distinction

Legal Framework

The legal framework within which home nursing must be developed remained limited. The significant rulings include the following:

1. Royal Decree of December 27, 1950, promoting the family activity of services providing home nursing. This decree, which has now been repealed, instituted grants for recognized home nursing subsidies. As a consequence of the new legislation, services for home nursing have been replaced by home nursing teams and cooperation initiatives.
2. A national agreement between registered nurses, midwives, certified nurses, nursing aides, and health insurance funds now exists. This agreement, formed between the health insurance funds and nurses' unions, was first ratified in March 1964 by the National Institute for Health Insurance (INAMI). It describes the relationships between nurses and insured people, as far as the fees and their means of payment are concerned. The fees are due for all nursing activities mentioned in the list defined in a Royal Decree. These financial guidelines have far-reaching consequences for the organization and operation of home nursing. A new regulation was instituted in April 1991, under which a set fee was introduced, in addition to the fee per activity, for home nursing clients requiring extended care.

   The Katz scale is used to assess this "extended care." This means that the nurse must now describe the patient's need for care with respect to six variables that include the "activities of daily life." A link has been established between the refund system and the need for care. In addition, the Flemish and Walloon communities have organized their own guidelines for multidisciplinary cooperation.

FROM HOME NURSING TO AID AND ASSISTANCE AT HOME

According to the World Health Organization (WHO), there is more to health than simply the absence of illness. It includes physical, psychological, and social well-being. This currently universally accepted definition makes it clear that taking care of health at home is a complex issue, which, in addition to the intervention of the general practitioner and the nurse, may also rely on domestic and geriatric help as well as social and other services.

DOMESTIC AND GERIATRIC HELP SERVICES

Services for domestic and geriatric help came into being after World War II and were established by private charitable institutions. A Regent's Decree of March 1, 1949, organized grants for home help services. Two decrees, published in 1965, describe the status of domestic and geriatric help and have had an impact on the evolution of these services. These services aim at providing temporary help to families and older or handicapped people who, for physical or mental reasons, are unable to fulfill their domestic activities. During the assistance process, the caregiver must focus on the person as a whole, remembering his or her desire to continue living in their own home.

Functioning and Organization

Assistance is provided by registered domestic and geriatric help services. A social worker monitors the work of these services and is responsible for the social study of the request. This must, in principle, always precede the assistance itself and the adjustments made to the assistance in accordance with emergency situations.

The provided help is temporary in nature. The aim is to restore the patient's *independence*. The possibility of turning to relatives or neighbors for help is also considered. A decree of June 22, 1988, deals with the recognition of and grants to services, training centers, and the statute of caregivers. The main recognition criteria to be met by the services are (a) being established by the local social services or by a nonprofit association; (b) employing at least three care providers; (c) applying the new providers' status; (d) employing one social worker per 150 serviced families; and (e) hiring one department head per 150 providers.

New services are registered only when there is a need evidenced by a survey. The principle is that the assistance must benefit as many people as possible. Strict limits were maintained under the previous legislation: 3 months of intensive help and then a maximum of 16 hours per week. The current legislation makes a distinction between the two periods of care: (a) an unrestricted period of 13 weeks and (b) then a period restricted to 32 hours per week. The assistance can be provided between 7 A.M. and 8 P.M., and at times when the need is highest.

Assistance is provided to all needy people, irrespective of their political, religious, or philosophical affiliation. Priority is given to the most needy and financially deprived people. The patient, family, doctor, or social services can simply contact these services in writing or by telephone.

The services offered include the following: domestic activities (meals, cleaning, ironing, sewing and repairing, and maintaining the house); nursing activities (helping with the daily or weekly toilet, preparing diet food, and taking care of medication); maintaining the family ties and spirit (welcoming children and looking after them and creating contacts with children, family, and neighbors); miscellaneous contacts (administration, bank, post office, health insurance fund, shopping, and referrals to institutions); and psychological help (listening, moral support, preparation of admission to an institution, terminal care, etc.).

Families, older and handicapped people are responsible for an hourly rate, which varies in accordance with the income and the family structure. These rates are determined by the community minister.

SOCIAL WELFARE INSTITUTIONS

In Belgium, social welfare is organized through the municipal social services (Public Center for Social Welfare) or through the Center for Social Services. The latter includes centers that belong to the health insurance funds and independent centers.

As recognized Social Welfare Services, the services are open to anyone facing an emergency situation. If necessary or helpful, a person can be further referred to other services or institutions. People with health problems often face other difficulties. The illness of a relative has an impact on the whole family and is coupled with financial and professional difficulties as well as tensions at home. These needs are the reasons why the social welfare institutions have a job to do in providing assistance at home.

The following services are offered:

- Psychosocial guidance in accepting or learning to live with illness or handicap. This guidance is tailored both to the patient and his or her environment.
- Provision of information about social legislation (e.g., health insurance, replacement income, family allowances for the handicapped and orphans, all sorts of exemptions, etc.).
- Responsibility of a mediator, in applying for financial allowances and tax exemptions; in compiling dossiers for applications related to occupational illness or rehabilitation material; in the event of long-term (e.g., handicapped child or older person) as well as temporary admissions (e.g., holiday camp, specialized schools, or convalescence holiday).
- Referral to specialized services including family and consultation centers, municipal social services, judicial services, and domestic and geriatric help services.

In the health care field, the scope of services has recently broadened to include organized volunteer help working in cooperation with volunteers and professional caregivers. The service is offered free of charge, but the recipient must have paid the additional fee to their health insurance fund.

Meals-on-Wheels

The Meals-on-Wheels service supplies meals at home to families and aged or handicapped persons. The aim is to enable these persons to remain independent as long as possible. In 1991, 102 registered services supplied about 4.3 million meals. All services but one were organized by the Public Center for Social Welfare. The services were subsidized by another organization of social welfare.

Cleaning and Small Jobs Services

This task is complementary to the services offered by the two ambulatory facilities mentioned earlier. The cleaning service is called in when an aged person cannot manage to do his or her weekly house cleaning. Unlike the domestic and geriatric help services, the cleaning service consists of only cleaning help. The small jobs service helps with the tasks in the house itself or in its vicinity. The facilities spread in the beginning of the 1980s in a random and fragmentary way on the Flemish territory have now grown into full-fledged services meeting the needs of the population.

Those services, nevertheless, have not yet been subjected to any regulation. The aim is to integrate these cleaning services into the domestic and geriatric help services to regulate and plan them. A total of 275 cleaning services and 109 small jobs services were reported in 1991. Only 20 cleaning services and 9 small jobs services are privately run. The rest are coordinated by the Public Center for Social Welfare.

Other Services

Other complementary facilities (such as loan of material, personal alert systems, etc.) were created to support home care. Other professional disciplines may also be involved in home care (physiotherapists or speech therapists, chiropodists, etc.).

HOME CARE PATIENT

We drew a profile of the home care patient based on two surveys by the White and Yellow Cross. In 1991, data of 4,500 patients in four Flemish regions were analyzed. The largest represented age group was the 60+ year olds who make up two thirds of the population. A quarter of the population is older than age 80. The average age of the total population in home care is slightly older than 65 years.

Another survey carried out in 1992 on 7,000 patients in Belgium gives us an idea of the extent of aged people's dependence on care measured with the Katz scale. The need for intense care clearly rises with aging. The percentage of invalid persons who are highly dependent on others for their activities of daily life rises from 12% for the 60 to 69 year olds to 31% for the 90+ year olds. Conversely, the total dependence decreases from 61% for the "young" aged persons to 6% for the aged persons older than 90 years.

Three quarters of the clients calling in for domestic and geriatric help services are older than 60; one out of three is older than 80. The recorded data of the 1989 working year provides an overview of the Flemish community clients' file. It seems that a significant number of clients depend highly on care with 6% of the 60+ year olds meeting the criteria for intramural services. Eight percent of the clients older than 60 years need help with their daily toilet; 4% need help with eating, and 3% are demented. These findings illustrate how much more dependent on care the old-aged people are than "younger"-aged people.

Finally, the cleaning services' clients are nearly exclusively aged people, with a 75 years old average. More than 7 out of 10 clients are women. The cleaning services' clients are made up of people rather autonomous in the activities of daily life: Eighty-six percent were recorded as valid, which means a score between 0 and 1 on the Katz scale.

CLIENTS AND ASSISTANCE

The following questions are asked about the clients receiving services: (a) What is the portion of each group of clients per work type? What is their portion in the population? Groups include care at home, domestic and geriatric help, and the help of social workers. (b) What sort of clients are they? What are their care needs on the Katz scale and on the adapted Katz scale? (c) What help do the clients receive in home care? How much help do they receive?

Out of 3,850 clients in home care, 3,670 received care exclusively at home (95% of the clients); 72 (2%) received care at home and the help of social workers; 87 (2.5%) received care at home as well as domestic and geriatric help services; and 21 (0.5%) received all three kinds of aid. In other terms, home care has 93 clients in common with social work and 108 with domestic and geriatric help services.

The domestic and geriatric help services were made of 591 clients: 445 (75% of the clients) did not receive help from one of the two aid services; 87 (15%) also received home care; 38 (6%) clients received domestic and geriatric help as well as help from social work; and the 21 clients already mentioned who received the three kinds of aids represent 4% of the total.

Social work had 382 clients in home care: 251 (66%) only received help from social work; 72 (19%) clients also received care at home; 38 (10%) clients received domestic and geriatric help; and, finally, the 21 remaining clients who received the three types of aid represent 5% of the clients from social work.

NEW ASPECTS

This sector of care has been undergoing important changes in the past few years. These include changes in supply, organization, and the definition of care. The following new areas will undoubtedly experience future developments.

Palliative Care

Palliative care has been receiving much attention over the last few years. It consists of specific types of care for terminal patients given by a multidisciplinary team focusing on the quality of both the patient's life and his or her environment. The palliative team's most striking task often consists in combating pain. Care for terminal patients can occur in specialized residential units, in the hospital, in other institutions (home for the elderly), or at the home. Up to now, no special regulations have been developed recognizing palliative care programs. Yet there have already been impulses to encourage and support these initiatives financially. In 1992, INAMI allotted a budget of $175 million to finance palliative care. This allowed 70 initiatives to be subsidized.

Cooperation and Coordination

Older people wish to stay in their own environment as long as possible surrounded by adequate care. Achieving this tailored care supposes an efficient organization of care. It requires cooperation and coordination between former and future initiatives among professional carers, sociomedical actions, and volunteers' work. The appointment of an intermediary comes within this framework. The intermediary would be in charge of organizing care through consultation with the patient, his or her environment, and the professionals involved. The Flemish Executive's decree (December 21, 1990) concerning coordination and support of domiciliary care is an important and positive impulse that allows cooperative initiatives to be subsidized and helps to stimulate providers in domiciliary care. Presently, 60 cooperative initiatives have been registered.

CONCLUSION

Home care has already come a long way in Belgium. Aid and assistance at home have always existed and have gone through ups and downs over the years.

During the past 15 years, home care has often made headlines to a large extent because of a health policy focusing on economies and spending cuts in the intramural sector. Partly as a consequence of demographic factors, such as the important aging of the population and the increase of the so-called civilization illnesses, home care seemed to be a formula that adequately fit the people's needs.

Home care will undoubtedly have to improve its distinctive features against the background of a global health care policy. More intensive relationships must be built, the gap in intramural care must be bridged, the preventative aspect of primary health care must be further developed, professional and volunteer help must improve their cohesion, and the goal of patient independence must further be emphasized in professional help.

Within the context of the global care policy in Belgium, the White and Yellow Cross tries, in alliance with doctors' associations, to obtain *scaling*[1] of health care. This is a necessary condition to achieve a better run health care system. These are the challenges for the coming years.

---

[1] Scaling means dividing health care in steps. The first step, primary health care, includes home care and the home-replacing sphere (e.g., nursing homes). Primary health care is close to the patient, there is permanent access, and it is provided by polyvalent carers. The second step, secondary health care, corresponds to hospitals. It is more centralized, specialistic, and intermittent (in casu "organ oriented" [heart, kidneys, etc.]). Both steps so much differ from one another and are so complementary that the disappearance of the limits between the two is damaging for the quality and increases the cost.

REFERENCES

Annual Report (1993), (1994), White and Yellow Cross. Brochure d'information (1993). La Croix Jaune et Blanche.

Vandenbroele, H., Bode, A., Leus, I., & van Loon, H. (1993). *The screening of clients in home care.* White and Yellow Cross.

CHAPTER 7

Ambulatory Care in Germany

Martin Moers
(translated by Ursula Springer, PhD)

Two major trends contribute to the growing need for ambulatory care in the German health care system. One is the demographic increase of the older population; the other, related to population aging, is the growing preponderance of chronic diseases. In addition to the usual nursing and medical cases, chronic disease cases require counseling, rehabilitative care, and social services. These problems usually strain and often surpass the human resources of families, especially since (a) women—traditional caregivers—nowadays tend to work outside the home, or (b) there is no family available for eldercare.

To provide the needed services in health care as well as deal with social or daily living problems, lay helpers (family or friends) usually supplement the services of professionals (nurses, doctors, etc.). This combination of lay caregiving and professional work is a growing phenomenon that calls for new concepts and efforts to strengthen the efficacy of the services.

As a result, the *Sozialstation*—social center—was born, a novel entity in German society. The purpose of these new centers was mainly the coordination of services supplied by charitable and religious organizations, the Red Cross, etc., as well as by local or state governmental agencies (hospitals, social welfare, etc.). The more systematic planning and avoidance of duplication of work resulted in a certain amount of savings and a more rational allocation of resources. From a health policy perspective, the new social centers were also intended to reverse the trend toward institutionalization, as the emphasis was to be on home care.

A social center is a community agency, based on local initiative, with financial support from the state government (not the federal government). The administrative work is handled by local charitable associations, including the Catholic charities, the Protestant diaconate, the Red Cross, the workers welfare organizations, sometimes the Johanniter aid service, and others. In some cases, mostly in rural areas, the communities (town or village) are the administrators.

The first models of social centers started their work in Worms and Trier in the Rhineland in 1970 (Heinemann-Koch, de Rijke, & Schachtner, 1985). The experiment turned out to be very successful and other lands followed suit. Among the slowest were the two city-states of Berlin and Hamburg, but they eventually opened enough centers to saturate the area. In the mid-80s the phase of countrywide implementation was completed. About 1,600 social stations existed in 1987, and in the early 1990s the number grew to about 1,700. At the same time the number of professionals working in ambulatory care increased noticeably (to 21,894 full-time equivalencies, but still representing barely 5% of the total work force in nursing and health care (Höft-Dzemski, 1987)).

ACCOMPLISHMENTS AND LIMITATIONS
OF SOZIALSTATION

According to its original concept of coordinating health and social services, the social center has to provide home health care, elder care, and family care as well as community services in a broad sense. In addition, other health services like physiotherapy, podiatry, rehabilitation as well as social services like transportation, housework, meals-on-wheels, visitors, and library services were to be provided. The main goal was to help persons in need of care in their homes. Another purpose was the activation of self-help and neighborly help. The social center was to become a meeting place in the community. Initially, some centers planned to provide a certain amount of ambulatory care on the premises; main activities were to be counseling and referrals. Counseling was to include spiritual and social counseling, family, marriage, educational counseling, and even psychotherapy, if needed. To activate self-help, courses in home care, neighborhood care, and medical technology were to be offered. The traditional "visiting nurses" were to be integrated with newly employed nurses whose 3-year training would guarantee the quality of ambulatory care that would relieve the hospitals from excessive use.

Resistance to this comprehensive model of a *Sozialstation* came from some religious congregations or parishes that took a dim view of the fact that the congregational or parish nurse would no longer work in her traditional role as spiritual caregiver. Some resistance also came from physicians who feared that certain medical functions (like injections, wound dressing), traditionally provided in doctors' offices, would now be offered by the social centers (Grunow, Hegner, Lempert, & Dahme, 1979). But the physicians' objections soon vanished. The social centers never turned into treatment centers.

Because the social centers, already in their initial phase, were over-burdened with requests and tasks, they soon reached the limits of their capacity. Most in demand was home health care, while social services and activation of self-help and neighborhood help remained minimal, with differences in the various regions.

As a consequence, the psycho-social, spiritual, and related dimensions of typical community care decreased, and the medical and nursing-care dimensions grew, sometimes to the limits of available resources (Stiefel, 1987). The goal of creating community centers in the neighborhoods was never attained. In the course of time, the social centers provided private nursing care in the old sense and gave up on community involvement. The separation of medical from social care thus continued to be strong.

One explanation of the turn of events was the rather small amount of resources available to the social dimensions of the planned functions and the fact that in social political discussions the term *central tasks* (Kernangebot) of the social center quickly gained currency (Forum Sozialstation Nr. 6, 1979). The charitable agencies agreed with the limited concept. And some later attempts at broadening the spectrum of tasks, like the provision of ambulatory psychiatry, drug treatments, or counseling, met with resistance, and never quite succeeded.

PRIVATE HOME CARE

Private home care expanded to the extent that the model *ambulatory before inhospital* led the insurance companies to include payment for home care. Federal legislation to promote this trend contributed to the financial bases of insurance—paid home care. Not included were household services at home.

The increasing need for home health care led to the growth of private home health service agencies. The first of these businesses emerged in 1984, working independently for social stations and were, of course, profit oriented. Some observers attribute the success of these private services to the limited capacities of the social centers, and the prompt services of the private agencies.

FEDERAL HEALTH POLICY
CHANGING COURSE

In view of the limited capacities of social centers and the growing needs of the aging population, federal initiative responded to the overburdening of hospitals and shortages of home care facilities. The topic of lively debates was the long-term care risks, and the financial means required to support such cases, aside from medical treatment. The discussions focused both on the need for long-term care insurance and the need to provide cost-effective care.

At this point, attention turned again to the social centers and their mainly medically oriented work. A statement made in the Bundestag (Federal Legislature) pointed out: "The ambulatory services, largely because of financial shortcomings, do not sufficiently meet the needs of those requiring care." A model program was established: Ambulatory Services for Persons in Need of Care. Fifteen social centers each received two trained eldercare professionals and up to 10 civilian volunteers (young persons electing social services in lieu of military service). The main goal was no longer home health care to avoid hospital care, but the avoidance or postponement of transfer to a nursing home. Since people usually prefer to stay home, the new emphasis combined humanitarian with financial goals.

Responsible for home care were the family members. Government intended to supply financial incentives to enable the family to do the job. The course of the model cases was successful. The volunteers for the social services have become indispensable. In the long run, the success is uncertain because of the manpower problems (where civil service volunteers are not available) and the ever-rising need for service (Brandt, Göpfert-Divvier, & Schweikart, 1992).

Additional problems arise from shorter stays in hospitals that discharge people sicker than in the past, thus forcing social centers to provide staffing for nursing/medical care that had always been a hospital function (catheterizing, infusion, difficult wound dressing, etc.). Also, the number and severity of chronic cases increased in diseases such as Parkinson's, strokes, M.S., cancer, etc., all now to be cared for at home instead of in the hospital (Brandt et al., 1992). The problems related to these long-term care tasks seemed hardly manageable by the social center staffs, who were trained to provide nursing care but not on the levels of severity and long-time needs as now appears necessary. The nursing staffs expressed misgivings at the demands made on them inasmuch as their training had not included the home and community dimensions of the severe chronic cases that are now referred to their responsibility.

Scientific analysts of the present situation recommend that training concepts be designed for new staff that include services and care of seriously ill people who wish to stay and die at home. In addition, the social centers need to be better equipped for these tasks. Communication and cooperation with patients and families need to be strengthened. Case management should be examined, as well as the initiation of care teams composed of professionals with family and other lay helpers.

REFERENCES

Brandt, F., Göpfert-Divvier, W., & Schweikart, R. (1992). *Ambulante Dienste für Pflegebedürftige*. Studie im Auftrag des BMFuS. Schriftenreihe des BMFuS, Bd. 6.1. Stuttgart.

Forum Sozialstation, Nr. 6 (1979). Unser Land bleibt Pionier. Interview mit dem rheinland-pfälzischen Sozialminister Gölter.

Grunow, D., Hegner, F., Lempert, J., & Dahme, H.-J. (1979). *Sozialstationen.* Analysen und Materialien zur Neuorganisation ambulanter Sozial- und Gesundheitsdienste (p. 68). Bielefeld.

Heinemann-Koch, M., de Rijke, J., & Schachtner, C. (1985). *Alltag im Alter.* Über Hilfebedürftigkeit und Sozialstation (p. 90). Frankfurt/Main, New York.

Höft-Dzemski, R., (1987). *Bestandsaufnahme der ambulanten sozialpflegerischen Dienste* (Kranken- und Altenpflege, Haus- und Familienpflege) im Bundesgebiet (p. 69). Deutscher Verein für öffentliche und private Fürsorge. Stuttgart.

Steppe, H. (1993). Krankenpflege ab 1933. *Krankenpflege im Nationalsozialismus* (7th ed.) 61-85. Frankfurt/Main.

Stiefel, M.-L. (1987). *Verbesserung der gesundheitlichen und pflegerischen Versorgung im häuslichen Lebenszusammenhang.* Bestandsaufnahme zum Förderungsbedarf (p. 88). Hg. von der Robert Bosch Stiftung, Stuttgart.

BIBLIOGRAPHY

Damkowsky, W., Görres, S., & Luckey, K. (1988). *Sozialstationen.* Konzept und Praxis eines Modells ambulanter Versorgung. Frankfurt/New York.

Garms-Homolová, V., & Schaeffer, D. (1992). *Versorgung alter Menschen.* Sozialstationen zwischen wachsendem Bedarf und Restriktionen. Freiburg.

Jansen, B., & v. Kardorf, E. (1994). *Pflege für die Pflegenden.* Modellprojekt des evangelischen diakonievereins ROTH e.V. Forschungsbericht. Institut für Gerontologische Forschung, e.V. München.

Trojan, A., Waller, H. (Ed.) (1980). *Gemeindebezogene Gesundheitssicherung.* München.

CHAPTER 8

Home Nursing in The Netherlands: An Overview

Ada Kerkstra

There has been a tradition of home nursing in The Netherlands for more than a century. In 1875, 10 local home nursing organizations were established. The tasks of these Cross Associations, as they were called, was to combat epidemic diseases and to protect the population from the spread of diseases by disinfecting clothes, furniture, and houses. They also lent material such as beds and blankets to their members (Kerkstra, 1989).

Several organizational changes have occurred in the last decades. In the early 1980s, there was a shift in governmental policy from specialist and residential care toward home care and primary health care. As a consequence, from 1980 to 1986 the budget of the Cross Associations was allowed to grow by 4% each year. From 1986 onward, the allowable increase was fixed at 2%. This policy has had some impact on the quantitative development of community nursing personnel. However, since 1988, the budget was reduced again (Kerkstra, 1989).

From 1980 onward, a compulsory public insurance scheme based on the General Act on Exceptional Medical Expenses (AWBZ) made it possible for everyone to obtain community nursing care, when needed. Since 1989, a large reorganization has been occurring. The number of Regional Cross Associations has been reduced from 160 in 1987 to 70 in 1990. In the new situation, a Regional Cross Association has a catchment area of approximately 230,000 inhabitants.

In 1990 the umbrella organizations for home nursing and for home help services were integrated into the National Association for Home Care. During the next 5 years, this integration also occurred at the level of Regional Cross Associations and the integration process is still going on. It is expected that this integration will increase the efficiency in home care and will avoid unnecessary overlap between community nursing and home help services (Ministerie van Welzijn, Volksgezondheid, & Cultuur, 1990).

Home nursing services include rehabilitative, supportive, promotive or preventive, and technical nursing care. In this chapter, the emphasis is mainly on the nursing of sick people at home. Other possible community nursing activities are not included (e.g., preventive mother and child health care, psychiatric care, midwifery, school health nursing, and occupational nursing).

ORGANIZATION OF HOME NURSING

Organizations for Home Nursing

Dutch home nursing care is organized on two main levels, namely, the following:

National level: National Association for Home Care
Regional level: Regional Cross Associations, 38
                  Home care organizations, 31

The *National Association for Home Care* is an umbrella organization for community nursing and home help services and has four main duties.

1. Policy making on the national level
2. Promotion of the interests of its members (i.e., the regional organizations)
3. Collective bargaining with government and insurance companies
4. Provision of services to the Regional Cross Associations, the home care organizations, and the home help organizations

As mentioned earlier, in 1990, the two umbrella organizations for community nursing and home help services were merged into the National Association for Home Care. At the time of this writing, this integration is still occurring on the regional level. In the middle of 1993, 31 home care organizations had already been integrated, providing both community nursing and home help services. The 38 Regional Cross Associations provide community nursing only.

Community nurses are employed by the Regional Cross Associations or by the integrated home care organizations. The Regional Cross Associations consist of several so-called basic units. In such a basic unit, a chief nursing officer (head nurse), about 10 community nurses, and 2 or 3 auxiliary nurses work in a team. A basic unit is assigned to a defined geographic area (about 35,000 inhabitants). Within this team each individual nurse, or a subteam of a few nurses and an auxiliary nurse, is assigned to a specific subarea. Most of the home care organizations have integrated teams in which community nurses, auxiliary nurses and qualified home helpers work together. In addition, there are separate teams of unqualified home helpers who perform mainly household tasks (Groenewegen, Kerkstra, & Jansen, 1993; Ministerie van Welzijn, Volksgezondheid, & Cultuur, 1994; Verheij & Kerkstra, 1992; Verheij, Caris-Verhallen, & Kerkstra, 1993; Vorst-Thijssen, van den Brink-Muinen, & Kerkstra, 1990).

Regional Cross Associations and home care organizations can be reached 24 hours a day and care can be delivered in the evenings, nights, and weekends if necessary. Patients are entitled to a maximum amount of nursing care at home up to 2.5 hours a day or three visits a day for an unlimited period. Patients who need more intensive home nursing for a limited period, mostly terminal care or patients who are waiting for admission to a nursing home, may make an appeal for additional home care. This additional home care is provided by private organizations or by foundations related to the Regional Cross Associations.

Because the Regional Cross Associations and the home care organizations are the main providers of home nursing in The Netherlands and also because there is no information about the number of private organizations for (intensive) home care, our description of home nursing in The Netherlands focuses mainly on the Cross Associations and integrated home care organizations.

Community Nurses in Home Care Organizations

There are three types of community nurses employed by the Regional Cross Associations or home care organizations (Adriaansen & van der Laan, 1989; Hingstman & Harmsen, 1994).

- *Community nurses* (*Wijkverpleegkundigen*) who have had either 4 years of higher vocational training or 3.5 years in-service training in a hospital with another 2 years of intermediate vocational training
- *Nurses in the community* (*Verpleegkundigen in de wijk*) who have had 3.5 years of in-service training in a hospital to become a registered nurse but did not have additional training in community nursing
- *Auxiliary community nurses* (*Wijkziekenverzorgenden*) who either had 2 years of in-service training in a hospital or nursing home, and a 6-month course in community nursing or 3 years intermediate vocational training in nursing

Community nurses are considered as first-level nurses and nurses in the community. Auxiliary community nurses are considered second-level nurses. Until 1993, most community nurses worked as generalists—that is, they provided nursing care at home as well as preventive mother and child health care in the child health clinic. However, the growing complexity and workload of home nursing affected the viability of working as a generalist. Therefore, since 1993, most home care organizations and Regional Cross Associations made separate divisions for home nursing and child health care. As a consequence, most community nurses specialized in home nursing or in child health care. Second-level nurses are only employed in home nursing.

In January 1993, 6,202 community nurses (4,353 FTEs), 2,017 nurses in the community (503 FTEs), and 2,933 auxiliary community nurses (1,854 FTEs) were employed by the Regional Cross Associations and home care organizations (Hingstman & Harmsen, 1994). In fact, there are approximately two first-level nurses (FTEs) for every second-level nurse (FTEs). In 1987, this ratio was 4:1. This means that during the last 5 years, the number of second-level nurses increased relatively more than the number of first-level nurses. In January 1993, there was one community nurse per 3,500 inhabitants, 30,294 inhabitants per nurse in the community, and one auxiliary community nurse per 8,219 inhabitants (FTEs). However, there are regional differences (Hingstman & Harmsen, 1994).

Provision of Services

In general, patients do not have a choice as to which home nursing organization they want to approach because there is only one Regional Cross Association or home care organization in the region. In some places, there are private home nursing organizations to which patients can turn. However, the insurance companies only renumerate the costs of supplementary home nursing under certain conditions and not the costs of regular nursing care at home provided by these private organizations. Consequently, the patient has to pay most of the cost himself or herself.

Patients can contact the Cross Associations or home care organizations themselves because no referral of a doctor is needed. Vorst-Thijssen et al. (1990) provided information on initiators of contacts with Cross Associations (see Table 8.1). Most patients appear to initiate the contact themselves, followed by those who are referred by hospitals or nursing homes.

Traditionally, the assessment is carried out by a community nurse (first-level nurse), who is also going to provide the nursing care or who delegates the care to a second-level nurse. In the Regional Cross Associations, this is still the case. However, most home care organizations, delivering home nursing as well as home help services, intend to combine the assessment of patient's need for home help and for nursing care. Within those organizations, there is much discussion about who conducts the assessment visits: a first-level community nurse who also

TABLE 8.1   Percentage of Patients Noting by Whom the First Contact Is Initiated

Initiator	%
Patient/family	47
General practitioner	17
Home help service	2
Hospital or nursing home	33
Other professional care providers	7

Vorst-Thijssen, T., A. vanden Brink-Muinen, and A. Kerkstra (1990). Het werk van wijkverpleegkundigen en wijkziekenverzorgenden in Nederland. Utrecht: NIVEL.

provides care, a manager of the home help services, or a member of a special assessment team. The fact is that the health insurance companies are demanding more standardized and objective assessment methods. By now most integrated home care organizations have chosen a special assessment team consisting of a few persons with a nursing background and a few persons with experience in assessing needs for home help services (mostly social workers). The members of the team make all the assessment visits and are not involved in direct patient care. This means that in most integrated home care organizations the community nurses are no longer entitled to make assessment visits.

The assessment forms used during the assessment visits differ from one organization to the other. There is no standardized form that is being used in the whole country. At this moment, new assessment forms are being developed suitable for assessing needs for home nursing as well as home help services (Verheij et al., 1993). At the integrated home care organizations, a member of the assessment team determines if the patient needs home help care. At a Regional Cross Association, a community nurse assesses the need for home nursing only. The nurse does not assess the need for home help services.

The same person who does the assessing also decides what type of care the patient is going to receive by what type of nurse (first- or second-level nurse) and during what period. Sometimes the member of the assessment team also makes a nursing care plan, but in most organizations the care plan is made by the nurse who is going to provide the care. Evaluation of the care plan by the community nurse who is delivering the care occurs regularly, but the frequency varies. When the care is provided by an auxiliary nurse, the evaluation is mostly done together with a first-level nurse. Community nurses and auxiliary nurses always work together in a team. In the home care organizations, they work in a team together with qualified home helps. About 7% of the community nurses are attached to a health center. They work in a team together with general practitioners, social workers, physiotherapists, and sometimes home helpers. Community nurses (first-level nurses) are qualified to perform all of the following tasks: assessment of the need for care; hygienic and other personal care (e.g., help with bathing, lavatory, and activities of daily living [ADL]); routine technical nursing procedures (such as injections, dressings, stoma care, and bladder washout); more complicated technical nursing (e.g., epidural anesthesia, handling respirator, and catheterization); patient education; psychosocial activities;

help and encouragement (e.g., from family members, neighbors, friends, etc.); and evaluation of care. Auxiliary nurses (second-level nurses) are also qualified to perform most of the tasks mentioned earlier, except the assessment of the need for care, more complicated technical nursing procedures, and the evaluation of care. In addition, auxiliaries more often provide hygiene care and less often give psychosocial support.

Client Population

About 5% of the Dutch population receive nursing care at home (5.7% in 1990, 5.8% in 1991, and 5% in 1992) (Landelijke Vereniging voor Thuiszorg, 1993; Ministerie van Welzijn, Volksgezondheid, & Cultuur, 1994). Table 8.2 shows the age distribution of patients receiving nursing care at home (Landelijke Vereniging voor Thuiszorg, 1993; Ministerie van Welzijn, Volksgezondheid, & Cultuur, 1994). The high percentage in the 0 to 4 years of age group is due to the health visits to mothers with babies and young children and is outside the scope of this study. Table 8.2 shows that mainly the elderly (70 years of age and older) receive home nursing. The number of patients per 100 inhabitants receiving nursing care at home declined during the past 5 years. However, the average number of home visits per patient increased from 8.9 in 1985 to 15.4 in 1992 (an increase of 8% every year). Especially, the mean number of home visits to patients of 70 years and older has increased sharply (Van der Kwartel, Delnoij, van der Meulin, & Harmsen, 1994). This means that patients of community nurses have become more care dependent and need more intensive nursing care.

According to a study of the National Association for Home Care, in 1993, 62.6% of the patients who received home care were females (Landelijke Vereniging voor Thuiszorg, 1994).

Relations Between Home Nursing
and Home Help Services

The relation and cooperation between home nursing care and home help services varies from region to region because a process of integration of both services is occurring. Consequently, in about 50% of the regions, home nursing and home help services are delivered by the same organizations; whereas in the other regions, home nursing and

TABLE 8.2   Number of Patients Receiving Home Nursing Care Per 100 Inhabitants

Age (years)	1990	1991	1992
0–4	40.5	39.4	38.1
5–19	0.4	0.4	0.4
20–39	0.8	0.9	0.8
40–59	1.3	1.1	1.1
60–69	5.5	4.8	4.8
70–79	16.3	15.8	15.1
> 80	38.9	36.5	35.3

home help services are provided by different organizations. It is expected that in 1996 both services will be integrated in every region of The Netherlands. However, during the integration process several problems have to be solved. For instance, the division of tasks between home carers, home helpers, and auxiliary community nurses has to be made more clear; especially regarding the ADL care because there is an overlap in the tasks of those care providers. Furthermore, cultural differences between the services have to be overcome to work together in an efficient way. Finally, many decisions have to be made about the new organizational form of the integrated organizations.

In summary, developments concerning the (further) integration of home nursing and home help services are and will in the near future be a topic requiring much attention in the organizations for home care. The parties involved continue working on the most effective organizational form for providing help/care to every patient or client.

QUALITY OF HOME NURSING CARE

Until recently, the government regulated the quality of care provided by health care organizations. The quality of care delivered by the Regional Cross Associations and home care organizations was regulated by AWBZ. Only health care organizations that are recognized by the Ministry of Welfare, Health and Cultural Affairs can provide care under this act (see also section 4.1). One of the underlying objectives is to guarantee a high standard of care.

However, the government now wishes to subject the quality of care provided by health care organizations to separate legislation, the Quality of Care Establishments Act (Ministry of Welfare, Health and Cultural Affairs, 1993). The Quality of Care Establishments Act abandons the principle of comprehensive central control. It is based on the principle of self-regulation. The basic principle underlying this legislation is that organizations providing care should themselves be responsible for the quality of services they provide. The authorities will adopt an arm's-length approach, although they will still be ultimately responsible. The act, therefore, contains a limited number of general quality requirements instead of a great many detailed standards and criteria. The aim is to create conditions in which quality is possible. The parties involved—health care providers, patients and health care insurers—must concertize the general requirements themselves (Ministry of Welfare, Health and Cultural Affairs, 1993).

The Quality of Care Establishments Act covers four key points that relate to the concept of quality, the scope of the act, the quality of the system, and monitoring (Ministry of Welfare, Health, and Cultural Affairs, 1993).

1. *Requirements for satisfactory standards of care.* This concerns the basic quality requirements such as an acceptable level of care (i.e., care that is effective, efficient, and patient oriented); sufficient qualified personnel; an acceptable standard of accommodation and equipment; and an annual report on their quality policy that is available to the public.
2. *Scope of the legislation.* The requirements of the legislation are obligatory for all types of health care organizations, as well as, for home care organizations and Regional Cross Associations.
3. *Internal quality systems—external assessment.* The emphasis is on an internal quality system that lends itself to external assessment. As the health care organization must itself assess whether the service provided fulfills the quality requirements, proper recording and assessment of the quality of care is essential. One of the instruments for external assessment is accreditation. If an organization fulfills the requirements it will be issued with a certificate. Such a certificate will also have a positive effect on the attitude of consumers and insurers.
4. *Monitoring and enforcement.* The Inspectors of the Public Health Supervisory Service will monitor the standards of care provided,

the way in which it is organized, and the way in which each individual organization monitors and promotes quality itself (the quality system). The emphasis is, therefore, on "monitoring monitoring." In the case of situations that pose a grave and direct threat to the health of patients, inspectors will have the authority to order an organization to terminate the care in question immediately. The organization will have a statutory obligation to comply.

A recent national representative study of Wagner, de Bakker, and Sluijs (1995) showed that more than 60% of the home care organizations or Cross Associations are implementing a quality policy and strategy. In addition, in more than 50% of the organizations, the managers use procedures to monitor whether sufficient quality of care is provided. The personnel (community nurses, auxiliaries, and home helpers) receive feedback about the results of the monitoring. Furthermore, around 60% of the organizations are implementing or have implemented quality assurance procedures such as committees on safety, accidents, and complaints handling. Also, patient satisfaction surveys are conducted, and the results are used for quality improvement. However, in less than 25% of the organizations, consumer organizations are involved in discussing the results of satisfaction surveys.

Finally, the Community Nursing Department *(Sectie MGZ)* of the Dutch Nursing Association *(Nu '91)* had ordered the Higher Vocational School of Nursing in Nijmegen to develop standards and criteria on community nursing. These standards and criteria concern the nursing care at home for ill people, the disabled, and the elderly; preventive mother and child health care; and patient education in groups (Peeters, Huisman, & Appelman, 1994). The standards are not implemented yet in community nursing practice, but the Higher Vocational School of Nursing has planned to conduct an experiment in which the implementation of the standards and criteria will be evaluated.

FINANCING OF HOME NURSING SERVICES

Funding of Organizations

The Regional Cross Associations and home care organizations are nonprofit organizations. Since 1980, about 85% of the costs of the home nursing services is financed through a system of public insurance based on AWBZ. The organizations receive a fixed budget from AWBZ, based on the number of personnel. They also receive money from membership fees (about 15% of the budget), which depends on the number of members.

For a Regional Cross Association (and home care organization) to be eligible for funding by the AWBZ, it has to meet certain minimum standards set by the Ministry of Health (Besluit Erkenningsnormen Kruisorganisaties, 1981).

- *Types of care that should be delivered.* These include (1) nursing activities in the home related to illness, disability, and old age; (2) mother and child care including periodic assessment of the child's health; (3) loaning of equipment; and (4) activities aimed at preventing illness and unhealthy habits.
- *Accessibility.* Twenty-four hours a day to be able to provide care in urgent cases.
- *Personnel in direct patient care.* One community nurse for every 3,450 inhabitants, one auxiliary nurse for every three community nurses, and one head nurse for every nine community nurses or auxiliary nurses. This standard, however, has become obsolete.
- *Quality control.* State employed public health inspectors have to be allowed free access at all times. However, since January 1994, the system of and the conditions for funding, are changing. Every individual regional Cross Association or home care organization has to make an agreement with the insurance companies and health insurance funds in the region about the conditions or standards for funding by the AWBZ. In such a contract the following matters are agreed on (van der Kwartel et al., 1994):
  - Prerequisites for delivering nursing care to the insured patients
  - Procedures concerning refusal or continuation of care
  - Right of reimbursement of the care by AWBZ
  - Standards of quality of care
  - Conditions regarding the registration of personal characteristics of patients
  - Information concerning the care provided by the Cross Association and the manner of control by the insurance company
  - Frequency and character of consultations between the parties

- Method of reimbursement
- Procedures in case of disagreement

Furthermore, from 1995 onward, the budget of a Regional Cross Association or home care organization will no longer be based on the number of personnel but on the "output" (i.e., on the amount of care provided). This means that each year a Regional Cross Association or home care organization has to make, in advance, an agreement with the health insurance funds about the amount of care that will be provided. In addition, they have to supply information concerning the care that has been provided during the past year.

Payment and Patients' Insurance

As mentioned before, since 1980 the Regional Cross Associations (and also home nursing provided by the integrated home care organizations) are about 85% funded by a system of public insurance based on AWBZ. Under the provisions of this act, all residents of The Netherlands are entitled to receive community nursing care, and no prescription from a physician is needed except for medical treatment. The remaining 15% are largely paid by patients' membership fees that vary regionally (average [NLG] 50; 50 NLG [Dutch florins] = $30.30 each year per family) because patients have to be (or to become) a member of the Regional Cross Association to receive nursing care at home. This annual fee can be regarded as copayment. The Regional Cross Associations and home care organizations are free to determine the level of the membership fees within certain limits. Cross Associations with higher membership fees can provide extra care or service facilities. Based on this AWBZ, patients are entitled to a maximum of nursing care at home up to 2.5 hours a day or three visits a day for an unlimited period (as long as they need help). In addition, loan of nursing equipment like wheelchairs, beds, and so on is free during the first 3 months. After that period, patients have to rent the equipment or buy the equipment themselves.

Furthermore, there are conditions in which additional home care can be obtained by patients who have a public health insurance, namely, when:

- Regular community nursing is considered not to be sufficient, for instance, in the case of terminal home care.

- Additional home care substitutes care in hospital or nursing home.
- The period during which additional home care is needed is limited to a maximum of 3 months. Only in exceptional cases is a maximum period of 6 months allowed.
- The total cost of the home care does not exceed NLG 410 ($248) a day (Ministerie van Welzijn, Volksgezondheid, & Cultuur, 1991).

The additional home care includes home nursing as well as home help services.

Also, nearly all private insurance companies reimburse additional home care, especially when the additional home care substitutes hospital care. However, there is great variation in the conditions for reimbursement between the different private insurance companies (van der Kwartel et al., 1994).

Payment of the Nurses

All community nurses and auxiliary community nurses employed by the Regional Cross Associations or home care organizations are paid a fixed monthly salary. In 1993 the gross salaries of community nurses varied between NLG 3,205 and NLG 4,246 per month (between $1,936 and $2,573 per month). The gross salaries of auxiliary nurses varied between NLG 2,827 and NLG 3,672 (between $1,713 and $2,254) (all on a full-time basis and depending on the number of years of experience and level of education).

Every 1 or 2 years, the National Association for Home Care negotiates with the unions about a collective labor agreement, which includes bargaining about the salaries of the nurses. In addition, most Cross Associations and home care organizations make use of nurses who are not formally employed by them. Those nurses are paid per hour.

PROBLEMS AND RECENT DEVELOPMENTS

In general, there are no waiting lists for home nursing care in The Netherlands. In December 1992, only a few Cross Associations had waiting lists, but the average waiting time was only 5 days. However, most of the Regional Cross Associations take several measures to prevent waiting lists. Four types of measures can be distinguished (Groenewegen et al., 1993).

1. Reduction of the inflow of new patients by using stricter criteria during the assessment visits
2. Reduction of the amount of care delivered to the patients (e.g., every patient receives less care than needed or the duration of care is shortened)
3. Reduction of overhead expenses or employment of more nursing auxiliaries instead of community nurses
4. Investment of the savings of the Regional Cross Associations

The increase in options for home care technology leads to the question as to what extent the community nurse is qualified to perform medical technical care. The division of tasks and responsibilities between nurses and general practitioners should be made clearer (Verheij & Kerkstra, 1992).

In many cases, the communication between hospitals and Regional Cross Associations or home care organizations could be improved. These problems concern the preparations for discharge and time continuity between hospital care and home care. Some Cross Associations try to solve this problem by employing liaison nurses who are based in a hospital and who assess the patients' needs for nursing care at home before the patient is discharged from the hospital. The nurse communicates these needs with the Cross Association to bridge the time gap between discharge from the hospital and aftercare at home.

Many community nurses are not enthusiastic about integration of home help services and home nursing care, as they fear a loss of their professional prestige. In addition, they fear losing their autonomy because of the introduction of special assessment teams. Finally, large cultural differences between community nursing and home help services have to be overcome. For instance, there are large differences in the level of education between community nurses and home helpers (Verheij et al., 1993).

Developments concerning the (further) integration of home nursing and home help services are and will be in the near future the main topic in the organizations for home care. The division of tasks and responsibilities between community nurses, nursing auxiliaries, and qualified home helpers have to be reconsidered and clarified to provide care attuned to the needs of the patients (Jansen & Kerkstra, 1993; Ministerie van Welzijn, Volksgezondheid & Cultuur, 1994; Verheij et al., 1993).

Regarding the funding of home nursing, in 1990, the Ministry of Health expected that the integration of home nursing and home help services would lead to an increase in efficiency in home care and in saving NLG 250 million per year. However, recent research has shown that until the year 1997, no savings could be expected from the integration process. From 1998 to 2002, a savings of only NLG 65 million ($39 million) per year has been calculated, and from 2003 onward, a savings of NLG 100 million ($61 million) per year is expected. This implies that less money will be available for direct patient care in home nursing and home help services than was expected (Homans & Glaser, 1993).

For 1994, the Dutch government reduced the budget for home nursing services by NLG 12 million ($7 million). However, NLG 20 million ($12 million) will be spent in reducing waiting lists in home help services and financing the change from care in homes for the elderly to nursing care at home (Ministerie van Welzijn, Volksgezondheid, & Cultuur, 1994).

An important development concerning the financing of home care are experiments, initiated by the Health Insurance Fund Council, in which personal budgets for clients are introduced. With the personal budget, clients can buy the care they need by themselves. The aim of these client-based budgets is to give the clients more freedom to choose the care they want. During the experiments, patients who were in need of home care for at least 3 months were offered the possibility for a personal budget. Forty-five percent of the patients chose this option. The first results showed that the personal care budgets can be threatening for the home care organizations because about 25% of the hours of home nursing care and 35% of the hours of home help care needed by the clients were purchased from private nurses or home helpers. As a consequence, if the personal budgets are officially offered in 1996 by the health insurance companies and by the health insurance funds as an option for clients in need of home care, the home care organizations will possibly lose a large amount of their budget, and as a consequence, will have to dismiss several staff members.

In conclusion, several policy measures (output pricing and client-centered budgets) include the introduction of competitive elements in the health care system. This means in the near future the advent of a private sector in home nursing.

REFERENCES

Adriaansen, M., & van der Laan, B. (1989). *Extramurale gezondheidszorg: Functies en taken van de wijkverpleegkundige.* Deventer: Van Loghum Slaterus.

Ministerie van Welzijn, Volksgezondheid, & Cultuur (1981). Besluit Erkenningsnormen Kruisorganisaties. *Maatschappelïuke Gezondheidszorg, 9,* 52–58.

Groenewegen, P. P., Kerkstra, A., & Jansen, G. A. (1993). *Wachtlijsten in de thuiszorg.* Utrecht, The Netherlands: NIVEL.

Hingstman, L., & Harmsen, J. (1994). *Beroepen in de extramurale gezondheidszorg [concept].* Utrecht, The Netherlands: NIVEL.

Homans, C. F., & Glaser, J. P. (1993). *Evaluatie integratie Kruiswerk en Gezinsverzorging.* Enschede, The Netherlands: Hoeksma, Homans, & Menting.

Jansen, P. G. M., & Kerkstra, A. (1993). Functiedifferentiatie binnen de thuiszorg. Utrecht, The Netherlands: NIVEL.

Kerkstra, A. (1989). Community nursing in The Netherlands. In A. Kerkstra & R. Verheij (Eds.), *Community Nursing: Proceedings of the International Conference on Community Nursing.* Utrecht, The Netherlands: NIVEL.

Landelijke Vereniging voor Thuiszorg. (1993). *Meerjarenraming "Thuiszorg in Beeld."* Bunnik: Author.

Landelijke Vereniging voor Thuiszorg. (1994). *Jaarboek Thuiszorg, 1993.* Utrecht, The Netherlands: NZI/LVT.

Ministerie van Welzijn, Volksgezondheid, & Cultuur. (1990). *Heroverwegingsonderzoek, Van Samenwerken naar Samengaan.* Rijswijk, The Netherlands: Author.

Ministerie van Welzijn, Volksgezondheid, & Cultuur. (1991). *Thuiszorg in de jaren '90: Brief van de Staatssecretaris van Welzijn, Volksgezondheid en Cultuur aan de Voorzitter van de Tweede Kamer der Staten-Generaal.* Rijkswijk, The Netherlands: Author.

Ministerie van Welzijn, Volksgezondheid, & Cultuur. (1994). *Financieel overzicht zorg.* Rijswijk, The Netherlands: Author.

Ministry of Welfare, Health, and Cultural Affairs (1993). *Fact sheet: The quality of care.* Rijswijk, The Netherlands: Author.

Peeters, B., Huisman, K., & Appelman, A. (1994). *Ontwikkeling van een kritisch kwaliteitsprofiel voor de extramurale verpleging.* Nijmegen, The Netherlands: Hogeschool Nijmegen/Nu '91.

Van der Kwartel, A. J. J., Delnoij, D. M. J., van der Meulen, L. J. R., & Harmsen, J. (1994). *Branche-rapport verpleging en verzorging: Feiten, ontwikkelingen en knelpunten.* Utrecht, The Netherlands: NZI/NIVEL.

Verheij, R. A. & Kerkstra, A. (1992). *International comparative study of community nursing.* Aldershot, England: Avebury.

Verheij, R. H., Caris-Verhallen, W. M. C. M., & Kerkstra, A. (1993). *Integratie kruiswerk en gezinsverzorging: Ervaringen van hulpverleners en clienten.* Utrecht, The Netherlands: NIVEL.

Vorst-Thijssen, T., van den Brink-Muinen, A., & Kerkstra, A. (1990). *Het werk van wijkverpleegkundigen en wijkziekenverzorgenden in Nederland.* Utrecht, The Netherlands: NIVEL.

Wagner, C., de Bakker, D. H., & Sluijs, E. M. (1995). *Kwaliteitssystemen in instellingen: De stand van zaken in 1995.* Utrecht, The Netherlands: NIVEL/ NRV.

CHAPTER 9

Home Care in Finland

Katri Vehviläinen-Julkunen

This chapter provides a brief overview of the Finnish system of home care, looking specifically at the way that home care is organized and at the challenges that the system will be facing in the future. Finland is the easternmost Nordic country, having 5 million inhabitants and a low population density of 16 per square kilometer. Most of the population lives in the south and west. Historically, the responsibility for providing health care in Finland has been thought to lie with the public sector. Since World War II, the Finnish health care system has been based on an arrangement where the local authorities are responsible for providing services and where responsibility for financing is shared both by local councils and central government. The health center system is designed to cover the entire population. Finland has 223 centers including maternal and child health services, local doctors' reception points, laboratories, local hospitals, and wards (e.g., Health for All by the Year 2000, 1987).

An important priority in Finland's welfare and health care policy today is to facilitate the participation of the frail elderly and chronically ill patients in their own care. It is considered important that the elderly, the disabled, and the chronically ill can cope as fully as possible in the safe and familiar environment of their own home. Home care in Finland is organized under primary health care, and its role within that system will continue to increase over the next few years. A central concern in the development of the existing service structure is to increase community care and mixed services so that most of the elderly population can continue to live at home and receive professional home care services.

Ultimately, the aim is to reduce levels of institutional care (Kananoja & Elovainio, 1994).

The aging of the population represents a major challenge to Finnish health policy. It is expected that the number of people at pensionable age relative to the population age 15 to 64 will double between 1990 and 2030. The number of the old-old and those most in need of help will continue to increase as the number of people older than 75 years is expected to increase threefold from the present level by the year 2030. However, there is a consensus of opinion among experts that the chief role of the public sector is to provide the basic services for the frail elderly who are most in need (Raassina, 1994; Vaarama & Hurskainen, 1993).

Under national plans for the organization of welfare and health care services in 1995 to 1998, programs for the development of community care are aimed at improving the quality of people's life. The basic principle is to listen to the individual clients and to respect their will. Where necessary, the functional capacity of aging people shall be supported through a wide range of services so that they can continue to live at home or in home-like circumstances. This support function is regarded as the chief role for old age services in the future, thereby allowing elderly people to lead an independent life at home, it will also help to give them a sense of dignity (Kivelä & Kivelä, 1985; Liukkonen & Laitinen, 1995; Raitanen, 1994). Home care services support independent living among elderly people and their ability to cope at home or in home-like conditions by providing care and treatment that is grounded in their own individual needs (Mäkinen, 1993; *Report of the Home Care Working Group,* 1994). Improved standards of home care will mean an improved quality of life and greater well-being for the home-dwelling elderly, helping them to maintain a good physical, psychological, and social environment for independence in old age.

DEFINITIONS OF HOME CARE, HOME NURSING, AND HOME HELP

Home care is a relatively new concept in Finland. It was coined in the early 1990s when the local organization of welfare and health care services was streamlined for closer cooperation. Home care consists of home nursing and home help services, which are complemented with various support and safety services as well as private help by relatives and voluntary organizations (*Report of the Home Care Working Group,* 1994). It can also be regarded as a formal support network (i.e., it is a form of care provided through the public system known as home care). Private home services and home nursing services are also part of the formal support network. The informal network consists of the significant others of elderly people, their spouses, children, neighbors, friends, and acquaintances. The help provided by voluntary organizations (such as the church) is also part of the informal network.

The norms governing home care in Finland are comparatively recent despite the long traditions of caring at home. The Primary Health Care Act of 1972 meant that earlier separate services were brought under one administrative and planning authority through the health center system, and that a uniform state subsidy system was set up to increase resources for primary health care. Since this act, it has been possible to allocate resources to primary health care. The services provided by health centers in large towns and cities must be adequate and matched to the size of the population. The goal is to emphasize the role of preventive services and community care. The Primary Health Care Act of 1972 obliges local councils in Finland to provide institutional and community care to their residents. Home nursing services form part of community care, defined as nursing and care provided at the client's home or in homelike circumstances. It is a systematic and comprehensive form of care that is provided to patients by the staff of the local health care center. According to the law, the home nursing patient shall also have access to all necessary medical and rehabilitation services as well as related health education. The guidelines issued by the National Board of Health in 1984 provide detailed instructions for the provision of home nursing. Home nursing is divided into supervised and other nursing services. Supervised nursing is more systematic by nature and involves the joint preparation of a nursing plan. Occasional home visits or home nursing are classified as other home nursing. The National Board of Health guidelines highlight the means and ways in which home nursing operations are organized and specifies ways in which they can be improved and developed. Although the guidelines do not refer explicitly to objectives, these include the continuity of care, security, service-mindedness, and an orientation to clients who have special difficulties coping with ADLs.

The concept of home help services was introduced in the 1980s. It was formally recognized in legislation on social welfare that entered into force in 1984 and defined home help as a universal social service intended for everyone in need. Municipal home help services currently consist of practical help provided by a homemaker and home helper, home help proper, various support services (Meals-on-Wheels, laundry services, etc.), and the home care allowance (a subsidy that is paid to a private person for looking after an elderly or disabled person at the client's home).

Most of the research on home care in Finland is concerned with the frail elderly. In the fields of medicine, the social sciences, and nursing science, research has largely concentrated on coping at home among the elderly as well as on home help and nursing services (e.g., Jylhä, 1993; Liukkonen & Laitinen, 1995; Raatikainen, 1992; Valvanne et al., 1991; van der Zee et al., 1994). There has also been a lot of work done to study the support that elderly people receive from the formal network (Kerkstra & Bremster, 1994; Liukkonen & Laitinen, 1995; Raatikainen, 1992; Vaarama, 1992). According to the results, elderly people seem to feel that the support they receive is more or less adequate, and that the quality of the service is generally good. However, there is also some criticism that staff members are pressed for time, that the care they receive tends to be superficial and focused on technical performance, and that there is not enough emotional support. It has also been widely observed that people expect to get more help from formal sources than they actually do. However, it is noteworthy that the amount of help that elderly people receive from relatives is 3 to 5 times greater than the help they receive from formal sources (Liukkonen & Laitinen, 1995; Vaarama, 1992).

ORGANIZATION OF HOME CARE, CARE PROVIDERS, AND CLIENTS

As we have seen, home care is essentially a combination of home help, home nursing, and support services provided for the frail elderly living at home. The aim is to support independent living at home or in a home-like environment by providing care and attention on the basis of the needs of the individual client. Distinctive characteristics of this work include the promotion of the client's functional capacity and independence, respecting the client as an individual human being, enhancing the client's security, providing comprehensive and systematic care, and working in close cooperation with the client.

Home care services are typically produced by a multiprofessional team including a nurse, a public health nurse, a medical doctor, an auxiliary nurse, home helpers, homemakers, and home help supervisors. The team is committed to making a joint effort in which all the professional groups involved work together as experts of their respective fields. Services are normally provided around the clock.

The biggest single category of clients consists of elderly people, but clients also include families with children, chronically ill patients, people with mental health problems, and disabled people. In the case of families with children, help will usually be needed in families where there is only one parent, in poor families, in families with many children, in families with a disabled child, or in refugee families. In all client groups, the priority is to provide home care to those who are most in need. In addition to care and attention (home nursing and home help), support services aimed at helping people cope at home include Meals-on-Wheels, transportation, and hygiene services. Client security is improved by means of emergency telephones, for instance. When possible, care by relatives is supported by providing benefits and helping relative caregivers to cope through various recreational activities, and facilitating the organization of care into set periods. In the future, voluntary work will take up an even more important role alongside public services.

SUMMARY

The need for home care in Finland is set to increase in the near future with the dramatic changes that are occurring in the service structure and, importantly, with the growing number of elderly people in the population. For experts and care professionals, these developments will bring important new challenges. Finnish home care is still very much in a state of flux as the integration of welfare and health care services that started in the early 1990s continues to gather pace and influence multiprofessional cooperation. For nursing research, too, this is a major challenge: The health care system needs to have constant access to reliable and up-to-date information on the realities of home care. Nursing research is well placed to produce this information on people's experiences of coping at home, the role of their relatives, and evaluation of different experiments with home care. The use of technological innovations will also increase in the future, and nursing science will have to work to produce information on this aspect as well (Raatikainen, 1992; Vehviläinen-Julkunen, 1994, 1995). New approaches and visions are also called for in education. The Department of Nursing at the University of Kuopio has provided specialist nursing education at the master's level since 1994 with the aim of improving expertise in primary health care. The challenge is to provide training for new experts in home care for the 21st century.

REFERENCES

Health for All by the Year 2000. (1987). *The Finnish national strategy.* Valtion painatuskeskus: Ministry of Social Affairs and Health. Finland.

Jylhä M. (toim.). (1993). Vanhuusikä muutoksessa—kohorttitutkimus eläkeläisten tamperelaisten terveydestä ja elämäntilanteesta vuosina 1979 ja 1989: *Sosiaali—ja terveysministeriön selvityksiä, 6,* H–. (in Finnish)

Kananoja, A., & Elovainio, M. (1994). Työalan kehitys—vaihtoehtoisia visioita. *Teoksessa Sosi-aali—ja terveydenhuollon työn tulevaisuus: Stakes:n raportteja, 150,* –. (in Finnish)

Kansanterveyslaki 66/1972. (1979). *The Primary Health Care Act, 1972.* Helsinki, Finland: Valtion painatuskeskus.

Kerkstra, A., & Beemster, F. (1994). The quality of assessment visits in community nursing. *Journal of Advanced Nursing, 19,* 1205–1211.

Kivelä, M., & Kivelä, S.-L. *Aktivoiva vanhustenhoito.* Tammi, Helsinki: Painokaari Oy.

Kotihoitotyöryhmän raportti. (1994). *Report of the Home Care Working Group, 1994.* Kuopio, Finland: Kuopio Health Centre.

Liukkonen, A., & Laitinen, P. (1995). Patients' behavior problems in geriatric nursing: A follow-up study in Finland. *Facts and Research in Gerontology Journal: Long Term Care,* 131–140.

Lääkintöhallitus. (1984). Terveyskeskuksen päiväsairaanhoidon ja valvotun kotisairaanhoidon järjestäminen (Ohjekirje 6455/02/1984, No. 5). Helsinki, Finland: Ministry of Health & Social Welfare.

Mäkinen E. (toim.), Niinistö, L., Salminen, P., & Karjalainen, P. (1990). *Kotihoito, SHKS* (Foundation for Nursing Education). Forssan kirjapaino Oy.

Raassina, A. (1994). Vanhuspolitiikka: Lähtökohdat tulevaisuudelle. *Sosiaali—ja terveysministeriön julkaisuja, 6.*

Raatikainen, R. (1992). *Self-activeness in domiciliary care.* Department of Nursing, University of Oulu, Printing Center, Oulu.

Raitanen, A. (1994). Vanhuus kotona: Ympärivuorokautisen kotipalveluprojektin ja vuorohoitokokeilun loppurapotti: Ituja vanhustyöhön. *Vanhustyön keskusliiton monistesarja, 1.* Helsinki, Finland.

Vaarama, M. (1992). Vanhusten palvelujen tavoitteet ja todellisuus: *Katsaus vanhusväestön elinoloihin, palvelutarpeisiin ja sosiaali—ja terveyspalveluihin: Sosiaali—ja terveyshallituksen* (Raportteja 48, VAPK-kustannus). Helsinki, Finland: Valtion painatuskeskus.

Vaarama, M., & Hurskainen, R. (1993). *Vanhuspolitiikan tulevaisuuskuvat ja kehittämis-strategiat* (STAKES Raportteja 95). Jyväskylä: Gummerus.

Valtioneuvosto. (1994). *Kunnallisen sosiaali—ja terveydenhuollon tavoitteet ja toimintaperiaatteet: Valtakunnallinen suunnitelma sosiaali—ja terveydenhuollon järjestämisestä vuosina, 1995–1998.* Helsinki, Finland: Painatuskeskus.

Valvanne, J., Juva, K., Erkinjuntti, T., & Tilvis, R. (1991). Kotona asuvien 75-, 80- ja 85-vuotiaiden helsinkiläisten toimintakyky ja avuntarve. *Gerontologia, 5,* 105–113.

van der Zee Jouke, K. K., Derksen, A., Kerkstra, A., & Stevens, F. C. J. (1994). Community nursing in Belgium, Germany and The Netherlands. *Journal of Advanced Nursing, 20,* 791–801.

Vehviläinen-Julkunen, K. (1994). The function of home visits in maternal and child welfare as evaluated by service providers and users. *Journal of Advanced Nursing, 20,* 672–678.

Vehviläinen-Julkunen, K. (1995). Health promotion in the families with newborns at their homes: Client's views. *Social Sciences in Health, 1,* 3–14.

CHAPTER 10

"Hospital at Home" in the United Kingdom

Violet Wagner

"Hospital at Home" describes the delivery of care in the home that would normally be provided in the hospital. In the United Kingdom, the concept spread in the 1970s from developments in France. Today, Hospital-at-Home schemes range from acute care, which prevents hospitalization or reduces lengths of stay, to continuing care for people with chronic illnesses. They offer benefits for health care providers and purchasers in more efficient use of hospital resources. Patients benefit in being cared for in their homes and communities. However, financial benefits to the health service may be offset by increased cost to patients and their families (Marks, 1991).

BACKGROUND

The most significant change in health services in the United Kingdom in the 1990s was the introduction of the internal market. This separated the funding of health care from the delivery of services, bringing a clearer link between cost and care through contracts. Technological advances have led to shorter lengths of stay through more day case treatments, minimally invasive therapies, use of endoscopy or lasers, advanced drugs, and radiotherapies. These advances have strongly influenced the move from inpatient treatment to care in Hospital-at-Home schemes. In the case of artificial nutritional support, the move toward home care has been directly facilitated by new technology, such as flexible fine-bore tubes and new techniques for endoscopy avoiding the use of anesthetics (Marinos, 1995). For patients who are mentally ill, learning disabled, elderly, or children, the move has been toward more care in the community. The National Health Service and Community Care Act, which introduced the internal market, also clarified the responsibilities of health and social service agencies for vulnerable groups. All of these changes have catapulted Hospital-at-Home from an interesting innovation of the 1970s to a mainstream service in the National Health Service of the middle and late 1990s (Lisa, 1995).

Until 1990, the Hospital-at-Home schemes in Peterbrough and Derby were the most significant ventures into this form of care. Although the concept was popular with managers and nurses locally and nationally, the medical profession was not convinced of their worth in clinical or financial terms. By 1995, such schemes are being delivered as part of the range of mainstream services in many areas across the United Kingdom. This chapter describes the way Hospital-at-Home has developed nationally and locally.

NATIONAL INFLUENCES ON THE DEVELOPMENT OF HOME HOSPITAL CARE

The National Health Service (NHS) and Community Care Act and the continuous reorganization in the management of the health service since its inception has set a tighter financial and performance monitoring framework. Regional Health Authorities, which were previously part of the planning structure for local services, have become Regional Offices of the National Health Service Executive (NHSE). Regional managers have become civil servants, with key functions of advising government ministers and monitoring the health authorities within their areas. The NHS continues to be publicly funded.

The policy framework of the NHS has been strengthened, with a clear move from hospital to community, from secondary to primary care. There is an increasing emphasis on clinical effectiveness of services in addition to the longer-standing concentration on financial efficiency.

Changes in the organization of medical training and work have meant that the length of time taken between commencing medical training and reaching consultant status has decreased. More consultants will be appointed. Junior doctor hours have been reduced from more than 72 hours per week to less than 56 hours.

Nursing has also moved on. The United Kingdom Central Council for Nurses, Midwives, and Health Visitors (UKCC) facilitated greater flexibility in the nursing role through its policy statement, "The Scope of Professional Practice."

In April 1996, the management of primary care services provided by general practitioners, dentists, optometrists, and pharmacists, and the commissioning of acute, community, and specialist health services will be brought together within a single authority.

The legislation has also changed the system of management of community care for elderly, mentally ill, and other vulnerable groups. Residential and nursing home care is funded through social service departments or privately by individuals. Although health services from NHS providers are free to patients in hospitals and the community, people receiving social services are required to contribute to the costs.

All of these changes are being closely monitored from the central NHS(E), which oversees the performance of health and social service agencies on aspects, such as waiting lists, waiting times for inpatient and outpatient services, financial management, and progress on the development of community care (with the Social Services Inspectorate). This close monitoring has increased the importance of Hospital-at-Home services, which affect these key aspects.

STRUCTURE OF PRIMARY HEALTH CARE SERVICES

A significant characteristic of health care in Britain is the well-developed primary health care system. General practitioners (GPs) provide treatment and care for people in the community and are gatekeepers to hospital care. Medicolegal responsibility for most health care in the community is held by GPs, whereas their consultant colleagues hold this accountability for patients in secondary care.

Community nurses, such as district nurses and health visitors, care for patients and clients registered with GPs, and the tendency is toward closer working within primary health care teams. A policy document called "The Scope of Professional Practice" (UKCC, 1992) has facilitated greater flexibility in the nursing role, allowing nurses to take on some duties previously carried out by doctors. Within eight pilot projects across England and Wales, nurses are able to prescribe a limited list of medications.

Social services departments are responsible for the social care of vulnerable people in the community. The importance of joint working between health and social service agencies has been reinforced by recent policy. People who receive health care at home often have social care needs that are covered by social service staff. Close working between social workers and primary health care teams, however, is still not widespread. This detracts from the success of Hospital-at-Home schemes.

HOSPITAL-AT-HOME MODELS

Successful Hospital-at-Home schemes have depended on their balance between primary and secondary care. The major professional input into all schemes has been from nurses, usually with a skill mix of qualified and unqualified staff. In the various schemes across the United Kingdom, the nursing specialties involved have included district nurses, pediatric community nurses, community psychiatric nurses, and orthopedic nurses. These nurses may be employed by hospital or community services. Medical supervision is given by hospital consultants or GPs, or a combination of both. Some schemes include close working with social service staff to deliver a combined health and social care service. Models of services may be described as:

1. Hospital outreach (e.g., orthopedic nurses working under the direction of an orthopedic consultant from a local acute hospital)
2. Community based (e.g., district nurses working within their teams with patients of particular GPs)
3. Integrated (e.g., district nurses leading teams including social care workers, under the direction of a hospital consultant, with patients of particular GPs)

All three models present challenges in coordinating care across primary, secondary, and social care. Successful schemes are those that manage the integration of hospital and community nursing services (Anand, Pryor, & Morgan, 1989).

DEVELOPMENTS IN SOUTH ESSEX

South Essex Health Authority is responsible for bringing health care to a population of 700,000 residents in an area covering 68,000 hectares. Services must be purchased according to population needs within a defined budget. The population varies from relative affluence in the north of the authority to pockets of deprivation in the south. The higher deprivation relates to a high elderly population in Southend, more children and single-parent families in Basildon, and unemployment and poverty in Thurrock. The health authority purchases health services from hospital and community providers and manages the services of GPs, dentists, pharmacists, and optometrists. Like other authorities, it funds Hospital-at-Home schemes with the aim of improving health care for its residents while achieving the objectives on which performance will be monitored.

Health Services

The Health Authority purchases health services from several local and more distant service providers. Developments such as Hospital-at-Home are invariably taken forward by the four large local providers.

Basildon and Thurrock Acute Hospitals Trusts
Thameside Community Trust
Southend Acute Hospitals Trust
Southend Community Health Services Trust

Hospital-at-Home Schemes in South Essex

Before 1993, the only local scheme that could be described as Hospital-at-Home was the Community Orthopedic Project (COPE). This was operated in the neighboring Barking and Havering Health Authority by Havering Hospitals Trust.

Within the South Essex area, schemes have been in the planning stage with the first schemes being implemented early in 1996. Factors influencing the development have included the following:

1. The health authority is required to reduce acute hospital lengths of stay and move patients through beds faster.
2. The transfer in responsibility for nursing home care from health to social service departments has led the health authority to concentrate its efforts on treatment, recovery, and rehabilitation.

In 1993 and 1994, additional funding was given to areas in and around London to build up primary and community care services to decrease the reliance on large teaching hospitals. The more deprived areas of South Essex qualified for support. Funding of £123,500 ($190,000) was provided in the first year to develop two schemes.

1. Community pediatric nursing teams in the southeast and the southwest (Basildon and Thurrock)
2. Acute 24-hour home nursing support team (rapid response team) for elderly patients in the southeast

These schemes continued with additional funding from the health authority for 1995 to 1996. A community orthopedic team for Basildon and Thurrock (COMBAT) is to be developed in 1996 to 1997.

COMMUNITY PEDIATRIC NURSING TEAM—BASILDON AND THURROCK

The community pediatric nursing team was set up by Thameside Community Trust to provide home nursing care for children suffering from conditions that would normally have required hospitalization. Specific objectives were to

1. Prevent admission to hospital
2. Reduce readmission rates

3. Increase the number of day cases
4. Reduce the length of stay from 2.92 to 2 days
5. Improve collaboration between acute, community, and primary care services

Children nursed by the team include those suffering from chronic diseases including diabetes, cystic fibrosis, asthma, hemophilia, terminal illness, skin disorders, or those needing traction, day surgery aftercare, or gastric feeding.

The scheme is staffed by 7.9 full-time-equivalent, qualified pediatric and general nurses. The patient's hospital consultant retains medical responsibility, although the GP is fully involved in the care. Local pharmacists are also involved in most cases.

ACUTE 24-HOUR HOME NURSING SUPPORT—SOUTHEND

In 1994, the Southend Emergency Admissions Study was commissioned by the health authority and Southend Community Care Trust. This revealed that 10% of the elderly people currently admitted to the hospital (20 patients a week) could have been cared for in the community with additional support.

The acute 24-hour home nursing support team was set up by the Trust to support elderly patients in their own homes during an acute phase of illness. The scheme provides intensive nursing and therapy support and the patient's GP provides medical care. Protocols have been developed to ensure that care is consistent across the different care providers for the relevant conditions. The service is run in coordination with the social care support services provided by the social services department.

The nursing team consists of a full-time, qualified nurse coordinator, 2.35 full-time-equivalent nursing staff, and 9.48 full-time-equivalent care assistants. The nurses manage the care of several patients, drawing up care plans and monitoring and supporting the care assistants. Care assistants deliver general nursing care and monitor the progress of patients, calling on the qualified nurses and district nurses of GPs when necessary. Night sitters are used to observe and help patients overnight to relieve the family carers as necessary. In 1994 to 1995, the team cared for up to seven patients at a time at a cost of £123,500 ($190,000). The annual cost from 1995 to 1996 is £247,000 ($380,000).

Between January and June 1995, 100 referrals were received from district nurses (45 patients), GPs (26 patients), the accident and emergency department (29 patients). Fifty-three patients were given direct care, which prevented admission to hospital. In an additional 24 cases, support was given to the patient's carer to prevent admission. Conditions cared for included chronic cardiac failure, falls, hypertension, pneumonia, carcinoma of the liver, chest infection bronchitis, transient ischemic attack, emphysema, gastroscopy—postoperative observation, diabetes out of control—respite care, multiple sclerosis, and rheumatoid arthritis—acute exacerbation.

Care was provided by the team in collaboration with social service staff, physiotherapists, occupational therapists, district nurses, and a private nurse in one instance. An average of 74 days and nights of care were given over the 6-month period. The shortest period covered was 2 hours of care assistant time from the nursing team over 2 days, with 10 hours provided by the night sitter. The longest was 755 hours of care by the care assistant, 35 hours by the registered nurse, plus 70 hours of night care by a night sitter. The episode included physiotherapy for the patient who was being nursed through a serious bout of pneumonia.

COMMUNITY ORTHOPEDIC PROJECTS IN ESSEX (COPE AND COMBAT)

These schemes, due to begin in 1996, are aimed at orthopedic hospital services at home for specific rehabilitation programs. COPE is a shared project involving Southend Acute and Community Trusts. COMBAT will be run by Basildon and Thurrock Acute Hospitals Trust. Both schemes will be aimed at treatment and rehabilitation of patients after hip replacements, knee replacements, and primary open reduction of fractures of the neck of the femur.

Teams consist of nursing, physiotherapy, occupational therapy, and community care staff in both schemes. COPE represents a closer integration of community and hospital orthopedic care, whereas COMBAT is more of an outreach service from the hospital orthopedic directorate.

CONCLUSIONS

Hospital-at-Home schemes in South Essex have not been in place for long enough to fully assess their benefits. They are, however, being seen as possible solutions to the considerable pressures of hospital waiting lists and the health element of community care. Acute care, rehabilitation, and recovery provided in the home satisfy both of these pressures. Schemes will continue to be developed or expanded and will gradually become part of the mainstream health provision. Savings on hospital budgets have not been costed but are thought to be substantial. These will be measurable as the scheme progresses.

The rapid response team has been well received by patients and their families. Thirty-one percent of patients were referred to the scheme by the Accident and Emergency Department during the first 3 months, and only 6% of these required subsequent admission to the hospital. Fifty percent of patients are discharged into the care of the district nursing team, with 21% to social service home care, nursing, or residential homes. In an area where elderly patients take up a high proportion of hospital beds, the team has successfully diverted 75% of its 100 referrals from hospital admission in its first 6 months of operation. Although the numbers are currently small, care for elderly patients in hospital is expensive, and the numbers represent significant savings.

Assessing the success of the community pediatric team is a greater challenge. Unlike the elderly care group, prompt discharge from hospital is not a major problem, and the cost of home care for children usually falls on the parents in time off from work or an inability to take up paid employment when a child is chronically ill. The scheme allows children to continue as normal a life as their condition allows and supports parents who wish to care for their children at home. A recent study indicates the need for a high level of support to parents caring for children with complex care needs at home (Jennings, 1994). A full assessment of the scheme needs to be done in collaboration with Basildon Acute Hospitals Trust and local GPs. The internal market has placed acute and community services into separate trusts, each preoccupied with its own viability. There is a danger of competition interfering with the collaboration that is so important with Hospital-at-Home schemes.

As a nursing development, Hospital-at-Home has not had much attention from medical or clinical effectiveness research. More critical research is necessary to establish both cost and clinical effectiveness of home care in the United Kingdom. In South Essex, Hospital-at-Home is expected to deliver benefits in improved patient care and waiting-list reductions. The next 2 years will tell whether these benefits are realized.

REFERENCES

Anand, J. K., Pryor, G. A., & Morgan, R. T. T. (1989). Hospital-at-Home. *Health Trends, 21,* 46–48.

Jennings, P. (1994). Learning through experience: An evaluation of hospital at home. *Journal of Advanced Nursing, 19,* 905–911.

Lisa, C. (1995, October). Home base. *Health Service Journal, 12,* 28–29.

Marinos, E. (1995). An international perspective on artificial nutritional support in the community. *Lancet, 345,* 1345–1349.

Marks, L. (1991). *Home and hospital care: Redrawing the boundaries* (Research Report No. 9). London: King's Fund Institute.

United Kingdom Central Council for Nurses, Midwives and Health Visitors. (1992). *The scope of professional practice.*

CHAPTER 11

The Role of the Health Visitor in Home Care Services in the United Kingdom

Jean Orr

This chapter presents an analysis of the work and educational preparation of health visitors across a range of primary health care settings in the United Kingdom. Traditionally, the United Kingdom has had several specialists in community nursing. More recently, as the care shifts to the community, this range of specialists has increased, and these have been identified by the United Kingdom Central Council for Nursing, Midwifery and Health Visiting (UKCC, 1994), which is the Statutory and Regulatory Body for the Professions in the United Kingdom as general practice nursing, community mental health nursing, community mental handicap nursing, public health nursing/health visiting, community children's nursing, school nursing, occupational health nursing, and nursing in the home/district nursing. The principles underpinning the work of nurses in the community are (a) the adequate preparation of practitioners who are accountable for their actions and who respect the vulnerability and primacy of all those who require care; (b) the provision of a quality and care-effective service; (c) the adequate support of carers; (d) the reduction of inequality of access or care provision; (e) effective multidisciplinary and multiagency cooperation; and (f) the cost-effectiveness of all policies and services.

Health visiting has its roots in public health and has been in existence for more than 100 years. The role has changed to meet the health needs of society, but the promotion of health and prevention of ill health are still the main aims of the service. However, there are problems in the maintenance of a service that is dedicated purely to preventive health, and this is a trend we see in many other countries. Nurses, doctors, and other health personnel are educated to care for the sick, and most highly skilled personnel remain in sickness-orientated institutions. On any given day, in many countries, most health workers are devoting their full time to less than 5% of the population who are in hospitals on any given day. This militates against the achievement of the health for all goal, which must be pursued by governments that allocate the health money, by educators who prepare the practitioners for the health services, and citizens who press for health programs that are accessible. In addition, nurses, because of their sheer numbers, can press for changes in the sickness system where the doctor is the gatekeeper. In most countries, only 5% to 15% of nurses work in the community setting (Mussallem, 1988).

It is important to look at some reasons why home care and preventive health services are difficult to get on the national agenda. First, it seems that the more privatized the health care system, the less emphasis is put on prevention. Second, the medical dominance of health care systems means that prevention gets a low priority, especially if it is carried out by nurses. Third, home care services are often for women by women and as such may not be seen as important by the policy makers. The World Health Organization (WHO), in a report of Women's Health and Development (1985), outlined the major problems facing women and stated that women carry extra responsibilities for health through their contribution to the health of their families and communities, both formally and informally. They constitute most volunteers in hospitals, self-help clinics, and other community organizations. They are, therefore, already providing a giant's share of primary health care and home care, and yet women are expected to fulfill these multiple roles while being the least educated and informed.

HEALTH VISITOR

The health visitor is a registered nurse who has undertaken a postregistration course at a university. The course covers the principles and practice of health visiting, sociology, psychology, social policy, and social aspects of health and disease. There is an increasing emphasis on clinical management, program and care management, and team leadership. The health visitor is the main preventive health worker in the National Health Service. The functions of the health visitor were stated to be: (a) the prevention of mental, physical, and emotional ill health; (b) early detection of ill health and the surveillance of high-risk groups; (c) recognition and identification of need and the mobilization of appropriate resources where necessary; and (d) provision of care including support during periods of stress, and advice and guidance in cases of illness as well as in the care and management of children (Council for the Education and Training of Health Visitors [CETHV], 1965).

In 1977, the following definition of health visiting was formulated (CETHV, 1977, p. 8):

> The professional practice of health visiting consists of planned activities aimed at the promotion of health and prevention of ill health. It thereby contributes substantially to individual and social well-being, by focusing attention at various times on either an individual, a social group or a community. It has three unique functions: 1. Identifying and fulfilling self-declared and recognized as well as unacknowledged and unrecognized health needs of individuals and social groups. 2. Providing a generalist health agent service in an era of increasing specialization in the health care available to individuals and communities. 3. Monitoring simultaneously the health needs and demands of individuals and communities; contributing to the fulfillment of these needs; by facilitating appropriate care and service by other professional health care groups.

The workload of the health visitor is determined in two ways. First, if she is attached to a GP, she is responsible for the caseload of that practice even if this is scattered over a wide area. Second, if she is based in a geographic patch, then she is responsible for clients within that defined area and may, therefore, liaise with many different general practitioners. Although most health visitors are attached to a GP, there are local variations to cope with local needs. The health visitor determines who and when to visit and accepts referrals from many other agencies, such as the school health service and social workers. In addition, she may visit if she learns of a family or individual in need. Unlike most other social and health workers, the health visitor provides a universal outreach service—that is, she visits families on a regular basis without necessarily being asked to call. The pattern of visiting is based on individual family needs, such as the birth of a new baby. Contact is maintained mainly through home visiting, and by the provision of clinic sessions and group work. The pattern of visits/contacts will vary from district to district and depend on individual family need, local community needs, caseload size, and local policy. As child health surveillance forms an important part of the health visitors' work with preschool children and their families, contact is often arranged to coincide with the requirements of child health surveillance programs.

The object of child health surveillance is to prevent disease through early detection of any problems that affect growth and development, and to promote health. Health professionals work in collaboration with parents to achieve this objective. Hearing and vision screening form part of child health surveillance. In some areas, there are school nurses who are totally responsible for the school health services, whereas in others, the health visitor has considerable involvement. In many areas the health visitor links the school to the community and encourages community projects of relevance to elderly people and those with special needs (Orr, 1993).

LIAISON ACTIVITIES

Health visitors, because they are visiting a wide range of the population who are not in contact with other health and social services, can identify people in need and are seen as being in a key position for liaison work including identifying women with social and health problems at antenatal clinics; following up antenatal defaulters; completing home reports preceding discharge for premature babies, children, and elderly people; checking home conditions and social reports for children in pediatric wards; following up visits for cervical cytology; linking with social workers or agencies in child protection cases; connecting with voluntary agencies, such as Women's Aid or Mencap; following up infectious diseases, such as tuberculosis or contacting patients with venereal disease; linking with the local Social Security office in response to claimants' requests; coordinating with local services, such as housing, public health, or social services; and linking with the local hospital for referrals.

The health visitor sees all social classes and across all age ranges. Traditionally, she is concerned with maternal and child health, but her role has been widened to include all family members and groups, such as the elderly and handicapped. She goes to the families in their own homes and gives support and advice on all areas related to health and development. A major focus of her work is health education and health promotion both to individuals and increasingly to groups, such as mother and toddler, school children, and women's health groups. There are many pressures on the health-visiting service to further broaden its span of work because of the growing emphasis on health education and the recognition of the importance of prevention. Such pressures include: the growing number of elderly people; the greater emphasis on shifting care into the community for groups, such as the mentally ill and mentally handicapped; and the increase of family stress because of factors, such as unemployment and family breakdown.

CLINIC WORK

In addition to home visiting, health visitors see clients at child health clinics and well-baby clinics. These clinics are attended by a community medical officer or GP for consultations, physical and developmental examinations, and immunizations. Mothers can have their babies weighed, meet other mothers, and have access to health advice from health visitors. Subsidized baby milk and inexpensive vitamins are available. In many districts, there are pediatric developmental examination clinics where health visitors carry out a range of developmental checks including hearing and vision tests. In health centers and health clinics, a range of other clinic sessions are provided in which health visitors may be involved. These include well-women, family-planning, audiology session, ophthalmology, elderly screening, and child guidance clinics. The pattern of health visiting varies according to local health needs and size of caseloads. Health visitor caseloads have been traditionally described in terms of the number of infant health cards they hold (between 150 to 900), but increasingly this is changing, and recognition is given to the work of the health visitor with other groups. A study by Drennan (1986) of 130 district health authorities showed that health visitors are involved in a wide range of community initiatives. These fall into eight categories: (a) health campaigns; (b) health screening schemes; (c) the formation of, or representation for, special-interest or pressure groups, which covered a wide range of groups (e.g., Tenants' Association, Sickle Cell Society, and Under-Five Resource Center); (d) provision of health information at local events, such as agricultural shows; (e) collaborating with other workers to produce information resources; (f) involvement in health education in the workplace; (g) use of local media for discussion of health topics; (h) participation in community development initiatives, such as unemployed groups, rape crisis centers, and neighborhood health projects. The overall conclusion of this study is that although some health visitors are involved in community activities, there are constraints imposed by large caseloads, lack of management support, and scarcity of accommodation and funding.

While the health-visiting service adapts to local needs and resources, the principles of health visiting remain. There are four principles as set out by CETHV (1977): (a) search for health needs; (b) stimulation of the awareness of health needs; (c) influence on policies affecting health; and (d) facilitation of health-enhancing activities.

Although the health visitor uses knowledge from her nursing background, she is not involved in practical nursing tasks, such as putting on dressings or giving injections. The skills used are essentially social and teaching skills, although there are some practical ones, such as testing a baby's hearing.

In assessing the individual and the family from a social and health perspective, the health visitor has to consider many factors. She, therefore, has to build up a profile of the family over several visits, considering changing circumstances and the developing trust between herself and the family members. First, the health visitor is concerned with helping individuals recognize health damaging behavior, such as poor diet, and motivate them to change that behavior. This can be a difficult task. Second, she is involved in providing or encouraging others in the community to provide services or start groups to meet health needs. In addition, the health visitor may have a contribution to make to local associations, such as tenants or mother and toddler groups. Third, she tries to influence policies that affect health, such as poor housing. This involves liaising with the local housing authorities to make her clients' needs known. In addition, health visitors can work through their professional organizations to bring these conditions to light.

FOCUSED INTERVENTION:
THE CHILD DEVELOPMENT PROGRAM

An example of focused work with families is being undertaken by the national Child Development Program, based at Bristol University (Barker, 1984). This program was supported by the Bernard Van Leer Foundation of The Hague. It is a large-scale intervention study that involves health visitors, and it focuses on altering the human environment surrounding the disadvantaged child during the earliest years of life. There are five basic elements in the study: (a) It concentrates entirely on influencing the immediate environment of the child rather than working directly with the child. (b) The principal and secondary caretakers in the child's environment, the mothers and fathers, have been encouraged to seek their own solutions to the problems of child rearing with help and advice, rather than direction, from the visitors. (c) The concepts and strategies used are simple, down to earth, and relevant to parents. (d) Large-scale and rigorous monitoring has been undertaken to assess the quality of the reported achievement. (e) Changes have been made to the structures and functioning of the health visitors involved.

The study started in 1981 by obtaining the collaboration of six urban health authorities in England, Ireland, and Wales; a total of 1,031 families were involved, with 1,051 infant children. These families were recruited by health visitors and were randomly selected from disadvantaged areas within the six authorities. The parents of 678 children received monthly intervention visits from their health visitors for periods of up to 2 years. The parents of the remaining 373 children served as controls for a comparison of the effects of the intervention. Five project interviewers carried out comprehensive assessment of the home environment and children's development so that all parents and children, both intervention and control, were assessed 3 times at yearly intervals. The intervention health visitors were given an initial 9-day training course and were seen individually and in groups for discussion of cases and for further in-service training in the developed principles underlying the project (Orr, 1992).

There are no set programs or formal lists of behavioral goals for either the parents or the children. The health visitors have been trained to approach parents flexibly, discussing with them methods of stimulating the development of the children and how to overcome any development problems. The visit focuses on seven fields of development, namely: (a) language, (b) social development, (c) cognitive development, (d) pre-school educational development, (e) nutrition, (f) health, and (g) general development.

Each health visitor is given a large range of cartoon material with accompanying guides covering these areas. Three of these cartoons are used as one of the focal points of the visit. The parents can study them in depth between visits. The health visitor completes a record of social and health conditions and also records the extent to which the mother has carried out the developmental tasks agreed at the previous visit. A new set of development tasks is discussed during the visit, with the mother/father being encouraged to put forward her or his own ideas for the coming months. The agreed tasks are recorded and given to the mother to remind her of what has been planned. Health visitors are encouraged to focus on areas needing extra stimulation; for example, if there is too little language development, activities might be suggested in which the mother regularly placed herself and the child in a natural situation, at a window for example, where intensive one-to-one communication can occur between mother and child as they watch the traffic and people pass by.

Following evaluation of the first phase of the project, it was thought that because of the many demands placed on health visitors by other work pressures, such as clinics and crisis intervention, some health visitors should be allocated to enable them to concentrate full-time on the support, education, and guidance of primiparous parents. In other words, one out of every three to five health visitors should see first-time parents, with their colleagues undertaking other family visiting and carrying out structured intervention visits to those multiparous families facing particular difficulties, and also taking on a wider public health role. The health visitor sees first-time parents antenatally and postnatally at monthly intervals (or more frequently if necessary in the early months). She hands over the family to the generalist health visitor colleagues at about 8 months. Up to half the families are kept on for a period (a minority for up to 3 years), if it is judged that they need continued support. When possible, families that are handed over receive every 3 months support visits from the general health visitors. Essentially, the health visitor specializes in working with new parents to the exclusion of all other health visiting duties. The main program content is the support and guidance of all first-time parents in the participating areas, and the subsidiary program offers support and guidance to a selection of those parents (in the same area) who are bringing up two or more children in the face of serious social or other problems (Barker & Anderson, 1988).

Features of the Program

The program is complex and wide ranging, and it may be useful to summarize the unique and important features of this work. The program stresses the importance of working with the parents and recognizes that the parents are the experts on their children. There is a pattern of regular monthly visits made by appointment. The emphasis is on the health visitor sharing responsibility with the parents and eliciting a more in-depth response than may be possible in a traditional visit. There is a recognition that although the child is the focus of attention, the health and self-esteem of the mother is also of crucial importance. The health visitor does not carry out ideas with the child herself, as this can make parents feel inadequate. There is a positive approach toward the child's development, and reasons are always found to praise something that the mother is doing. There is an emphasis on the idea of child rearing being a matter of enjoyment, a concept that is often missing in other programs that emphasize precise goals, tasks, and achievements, like some form of duty.

More Recent Developments

Two developments arising from the original model are raising important issues for health visiting. An evaluation instrument known as the Early Health and Development Monitor is now being used in nearly half of the 25 health authorities collaborating in the Child Development Program. This instrument has a twofold purpose: to assess the effectiveness of program visiting, in line with the unit's belief that whatever is done should be subjected to ongoing monitoring, and to provide regular reports on the most significant outcomes of health visiting in relation to the health and development of young children throughout the health authority (Barker, 1994). The monitor is used to gather a modest amount of information during a 20-minute monitor visit to the home each year; this information is recorded on a single card, which covers the first 4 years on a child's life, and the card is immediately sent in to the authority's central office for data input on to a hard disk microcomputer. The focus in the monitor's development has been on creating something that is relatively informal in appearance and yet fairly rigorous in the way it has to be completed.

It is worth noting that although the instrument was initially devised purely as a field tool for evaluating Child Development Program effectiveness, its primary function today is to offer health authorities, epidemiologists, and health visitors and their managers an easily analyzable packet of information on health outcomes at any level, ranging from across the authority down to individual caseloads.

A more continuous recent development has been the introduction of community mothers, who do home visits to selected families and make use of the same cartoons as do trained health visitors within the Child Development Program. They also use simplified visiting forms. The women are selected on the basis of being experienced and competent mothers, who have the ability to empathize with and empower others. It is also a condition that they have to be living on the same housing estates as the families they visit. The first community mothers program was set up by the Early Childhood Development Unit in Dublin 6 years ago. The community mothers are guided and trained by public health nurses. There are now 150 mothers, visiting about 1,000 first-time families a year. Recently, modified versions of this same program have been initiated in the United Kingdom within two communities. In one city, an Asian Parent Program has been initiated, using Asian women from within specific Pakistani or Indian immigrant communities, to do home visits using cartoons translated (and modified where necessary) into Urdu or Gujarati. An equally interesting development has been the initiation of a community mothers' program in a socially stressed area on the southeast coast of England. It is an area where visiting first-time parents is already being undertaken. The community mothers work with multiple families referred to them by the generic visitor colleagues of those visiting first-time parents; the families are selected on the grounds of their social and child-rearing problems. As the community mothers come from the same neighborhood as the families they visit, they have a street credibility that no professional could equal.

CONCLUSION

Appleby (1991) in a review of health-visiting services shows there is ample evidence that health visitor intervention is effective in improving child and maternal health and the health of other groups. Appleby highlights that the type of outreach service offered by health visitors is a service without stigma that reaches those most vulnerable in our society who do not seek help. A recent publication in the United Kingdom called Progress Through Partnership (Her Majesty's Stationery Office, 1995) outlined the likely impact of current scientific and technological advances on health and social services. There will be changes in modes of service response including the substitution of one professional group for another, particularly as care moves into the community. The report raises several questions that are important for the development of home care. The first one is that the increased understanding of the genetic and environmental origins of disease will result in the widespread application of probabilistic medicine at an individual level. Current public health measures and preventive medicine are based mainly on knowledge of factors influencing disease in large populations. The fact that risk is not individualized limits the public compliance with preventive measures. There is every reason to expect that the next generation will see the identification of more widespread inherited factors predisposing them to common forms of cancer, heart disease, mental illness, birth defects, and dental disease. At the same time, we are improving our understanding of the link between genetics, metabolism, environment, early development, and lifestyle in the epidemiology of many diseases. Although the future is exciting and dynamic, it is important to stress that within the context of the technology it is the individual contact between the patient and nurse that is at the center of quality home care services, and that is what we must strive to maintain and improve.

REFERENCES

Appleby, F. (1991). In pursuit of excellence. *Health Visitor, 64,* 254–256.
Barker, W. (1984). *The child development program.* Bristol, England: Bristol University.
Barker, W. (1992). *The early health and development monitor.* Bristol, England: Bristol University, Early Childhood Development Unit.
Barker, W., & Anderson, R. (1988). *Child development program: An evaluation of process and outcome.* Bristol, England: Bristol University, Early Childhood Development Unit.
Council for the Education and Training of Health Visitors. (1965). *The functions of a health visitor.* London: Author.
Council for the Education and Training of Health Visitors. (1977). *An investigation into the principles of health visiting.* London: Author.

Drennan, V. (1986). Developments in health visiting. *Health Visitor, 59,* 4–6.

Epp, J. (1986). *Achieving health for all: A framework for health promotion.* Ottawa, Canada: Department of Health and Welfare.

Mussallem, H. K. (1988). Preventions and patterns of disease. In R. Willis & J. Linwood. (Eds.), *Recent advances in nursing, prevention and nursing.* Edinburgh, Scotland: Churchill Livingstone.

Office of Science and Technology. (1995). Health and life sciences. In *Progress through partnership.* London: Her Majesty's Stationery Office.

Orr, J. (1992). Assessing individual and family health needs. In J. Orr & K. Luker (Eds.), *Health visiting.* Oxford, England: Blackwell Scientific.

Orr, J. (1993). The role of the health visitor. In P. Turton & J. Orr (Eds.), *Learning to care in the community.* Kent, England: Edward Arnold.

Stockport Health Authority. (1992). *A strategy for health visiting.*

United Kingdom Central Council for Nursing, Midwifery, and Health Visiting. (1994). *The future of professional practice: The council's standards for education and practice following registration.* London: Author.

While, A. (1986). The value of health visitors. *Health Visitor, 59,* 171–172.

World Health Organization. (1985). *Women's health and development* (Report by the director general). Geneva, Switzerland: Author.

CHAPTER 12

Home-Based Health Care in Hungary

Zoltán Balogh and Doris Modly

The health care delivery system in Hungary is currently undergoing major reforms that began in 1989 to 1990. The aim of the reforms is to restructure the health care delivery system and place more emphasis on primary health care and prevention of diseases. Under the socialist form of government, all Hungarian citizens were entitled to both health and social services. Services were provided in the past as citizens' rights; they are now reimbursed by the National Health Insurance or covered by private health insurance (Sövenyi, Szegedi, & Druskoczi, 1995).

The focus on primary health care requires different skills and higher levels of competency by nurses for effective functioning in the new health care system. They must assume new responsibilities as their practice moves from institutional settings, such as hospitals, to the community and into the homes of their clients/patients (Nánási, 1995).

The efforts to develop a coordinated structure for home care and home health services date back to the late 1960s in Hungary. The services include both home care provided through the social welfare system by social workers and home aids, and home health care provided by health care professionals. Home care encompasses social services chiefly for the elderly in their homes, whereas home health care is defined as health care provided by the family or district physician and by district nurses under the physician's direction, both in the patient's home and the physician's office (Sövenyi et al., 1995).

Teamwork in home care, as defined by European standards, does not exist in Hungary at present except in a few newly organized, mostly proprietary programs and a few governmental pilot programs. Home health care is provided mostly for elderly who are confined to their homes. Since 1993, this service has been extended to the active adult population, who, because of temporary disability, are unable to care for themselves or their families. Home care is provided partly by professionals, and partly by volunteers. To implement some form of quality assurance of the care, emphasis is being placed on increasing the number of educated professional caregivers including trained home care nurses who can form home care teams.

A home care pilot program was started in 1991 in Budapest's VIIIth District. The Hungarian Ministry of Welfare, with funding from the American Joint Distribution Committee and the United States Agency for International Development, developed and implemented this experimental program (Tomcsik & Dénes, 1993). The population in this district consists of many elderly and relatively fewer younger persons who are in need of care. Originally, the program focused on home care for the aged with an emphasis on their social needs. Based on the real needs of the population, however, the emphasis shifted to care for patients with chronic health problems and to rehabilitation of both the chronically ill and the temporarily disabled younger population. The goal of the program became the care of these patients/clients in their own home. The aims were to reduce high institutional costs and provide care in a setting more conducive to rehabilitation. Since the introduction of this program in the VIIIth District in Budapest, several similar proprietary home care organizations have been established in Budapest and in other cities of Hungary, with financial support from their local governments.

The Ministry of Welfare announced a request for proposals in 1994 for the development of home care services. In response, several small Hungarian home care provider organizations were formed with the financial support from local governments. The Harris Health Corporation of Texas submitted a successful proposal in collaboration with local governments in three different cities. Harris Health Hungary now has three functioning projects and is expanding its services. There are several other local examples, some initiated by entrepreneurial nurses in cities across the country.

In the VIIIth District pilot program, the home care team now comprises the following professionals: the family or house physician, the nurse, the physical therapist, the social worker, and sometimes the psychologist and the nutritionist (Nánási, 1995). The program was launched with two teams in late 1991 after thorough training of team members in geriatric care. These teams were, at first, closely supervised but after 2 months began independent functioning. Then additional teams were launched. In 1993, there were 18 such teams functioning in the VIIIth District (Tomcsik & Dénes, 1993). At that time, the teams had cared for 208 patients/clients. Of these, almost 50% were patients with chronic mobility problems, 25% were victims of trauma, and 20% had suffered cerebrovascular accidents. The average age of clients was around 70 years, and most (75%) were women.

At the conclusion of the pilot project, the teams continued their work under the umbrella of the local government, and in collaboration with social welfare and health care services. The goal of the program continues to be the care and rehabilitation of older and sick persons in their own home in collaboration and with assistance by team members. The team's goal is to involve both the patient and the environment in the facilitation of a smooth transition from hospital to home and bring the patient to the point of being able to care for him or herself (Tomcsik & Dénes, 1993). Consequently, the patient and family members become active participants in the caregiving process and become team members themselves.

This program has great significance because now patients can be cared for in their own home with the assistance of a team of professionals versus the often impersonal, poorly staffed social service beds of hospitals where they stayed if they could not return home alone. In the past, if patients did return home alone or to the care of unprepared family members, their recovery and rehabilitation were jeopardized.

The clients most frequently seen by the home care team in the VIIIth District in Budapest are hemiplegic patients. This case study illustrates the care of those clients and highlights the role of the nurse and the physical therapist. When public health statistics of Hungary are examined, it becomes evident that the leading causes of both morbidity and mortality are circulatory/vascular and brain alterations. Three fourths of these are of vascular/ischemic origin, and one fourth are due to brain tumors and trauma. For every 10,000 persons in Hungary, in 1990, 71.6 deaths were attributed to cerebrovascular diseases; in contrast, 29.1 deaths were due to cancer, 12.3 were due to trauma, 8.5 were due to gastrointestinal problems, and 6.5 were due to respiratory diseases (Ministry of Welfare, 1994). Among the alterations of the circulatory system developed during the life cycle, the most frequently occurring pathologies are atherosclerosis, hypertonic encephalopathy, and endarteritis obliterans. These pathologies can result in transient ischemic attacks, brain thrombosis, brain emboli, and brain hemorrhages. Lasting brain damage results from the last three.

In Hungary, the problem of care of hemiplegic patients after their release from hospitals has not been solved. Protocols for nursing care, social support, and mobilization are not systematically organized, funded, and carried out. Consequently, the rehabilitation of hemiplegic patients is difficult or impossible (because of improperly aligned joints and contractures). Following hospitalization, in general, patients are left alone with their problems. Even if the patient has a family that is willing to help them, the family does not receive any support from the health and welfare system of the country. With increasing numbers of families requiring two incomes, the availability of family members to help is diminishing.

The rehabilitation of the hemiplegic patient should begin during the acute phase in the hospital. If cared for correctly, the hemiplegic individual can eventually regain his work capacity. Through collaboration of the home care team with acute caregivers in institutional settings, attempts are being made to achieve some kind of rehabilitation and independence for the patient.

At the start of the program, a thorough assessment is prepared by the team to determine the client's needs and the interventions necessary. Criteria for short- and long-term goals are established for the care plan. These documents serve as the basis for evaluation of interventions. The participation of key team members is essential, especially the physical therapist and the nurse.

Specific activities that are the responsibility of the nurse on the home care team are defined as follows:

1. Inform/instruct the family how to care for the patient; provide practical and useful advice.
2. Assist with rearrangement of the environment (room/apartment) to secure the most advantageous surroundings for the patient.
3. Advise and assist with selection of the most important patient-assistive devices and their use.
4. Teach family members basic nursing care and consult with the family regarding future problems.

5. Teach the family proper alignment and mobilization of the patient while in bed.
6. Teach the family passive and active exercises, and eventually walking practice and support.
7. Teach the family to assist the patient with ADLs, dietary advice, and food preparation.
8. Teach the family simple speech exercises.
9. Provide emotional support for patient and family.

The activities listed clearly illustrate the wide range of professional nursing knowledge required for effective home care nursing. To function effectively on the multidisciplinary team, a basic understanding of the other team members' knowledge base and skills is also required. Complex problems that occur in the care of the hemiplegic patient can only be solved through collaboration of the whole home care team. Only continuing education and development on the part of team members provide optimum results. The rehabilitation of hemiplegic patients is an arduous process that requires collaboration of all members of the health care team. Best results are achieved in an environment that is familiar to the patient, such as his or her home, the place of function. Involvement of family and other informal caregivers in the rehabilitation process is also most beneficial, not only for hemiplegic patients, but to all patients who need home care following hospitalization, as well as those with chronic illness. It is important to expand home care services in the rest of the country to achieve better end results for patients with perhaps a lesser cost to the health care system.

REFERENCES

Ministry of Welfare. (1994). Principles of a long-term health promotion policy in Hungary. Budapest, Hungary: MEDINFO National Institute of Medical Information.
Nánási, J.(1995). The role of international projects in nursing. In *Opening the doors to home care nursing:* Proceedings Book, Padua, Venice-Italy.
Országos Egészségbistositási Pénztár és a Nepjoleti Miniszterium Pályázati Felhivása az Otthoni Ápolási Szolgalat es Hospice Ellátás Fejlesztésére és Tamogatására (1994). *Népjöléti Közlöny.*

Sövényi. K., Szegedi, G., & Druskoczi T. (1995). Home care, home nursing in Hungary. In *Opening the door to home care nursing:* Proceedings Book, p. 133, Padua, Italy.

Tomcsik, M., & Dénes, M. (1993). A jozsefvárosi kisérleti házi gondozasi (home care) program elözetes ertékelése. *Egészségügyi Gazdasági Szemle 31,* 360–365.

BIBLIOGRAPHY

Charness, A. (1986). *Stroke/head injury.* Germantown, MD: Aspen Systems Corporation.

Milliken, M. E. (1991). *Mindennapos betegápolás.* Budapest, Hungary: Országos Orvostudományi Interzet.

CHAPTER 13

Home Care Nursing in Korea: Case Study

HaeOk Lee, Ae-Ran Hwang, and Hea-Young Kim

With advances in medical technology, a changing social structure, and an aging global population, many changes have occurred in health care systems including a new movement toward early hospital discharge and home care nursing. In the next decade, the needs for home care and related services are expected to triple (Lewin-VHI analysis of NAMES [National Association of Medical Equipment Suppliers] data, 1993). Governments, health care professionals, and sociologists together must determine how best to meet the rapidly growing demand for these services.

Traditionally, South Koreans have counted on the services of wives, daughters, and daughters-in-law to take care of ill relatives at home when they were sick or released from the hospital. Now, however, those former family caretakers are at work. As South Korea grows more prosperous and Korean women leave domestic duties for jobs in factories and offices, a new problem has emerged for the society. Simply put, there are too few relatives left at home to care for the elderly and sick. In addition, the culture is changing. There's no doubt that Koreans are becoming Westernized, or Americanized; they are more interested in living in a nuclear family than an extended family. As a result, there are fewer families with several generations living together, and more women have jobs. Given the characteristics of today's nuclear family, the increasing number of women in jobs, and the increasing number of sick elderly individuals who need to be cared for at home, there is a critical demand for competent clinical nurses with advanced educational preparation to manage and facilitate the care of patients in the home.

The advantages of receiving care in the home are generally recognized. Not only is home care usually preferred by the older adult, but it is also necessitated by the costs of institutional care. However, we know little about the economic, physical, psychological, and social costs and benefits of long-term care at home for the family and patient. In addition, professionals in nursing need to recognize the strengths of families in providing care to the elderly and sick, and also begin to acknowledge the family's limitations.

CASE STUDIES

The objective of these case studies is to provide information about home care nursing in Korea in terms of the clinical, technological, psychological, financial, and social impact on two patients.

Case 1

A 48-year-old married woman had metastatic cervical carcinoma. She had a 2-month history of whitish vaginal secretions. This followed an abdominal hysterectomy with salpingo-oophorectomy. Her operational wound healed without problems, but she was retaining 150 to 200 mL of urine and was experiencing constipation. The patient thought that inadequate privacy for using the rest room with other patients and visitors nearby caused these problems. On the patient's request, she was discharged 4 days earlier than her scheduled discharge, after 18 days of hospitalization. Home care nurses were asked to assess the patient's condition for home care services before discharge.

This patient had two unmarried daughters and one married son. She lived with her husband and two daughters, all of whom worked during the day. Her son and daughter-in-law lived close by, and the daughter-in-law was to be the primary caregiver; she was active and positive in learning about the patient's home care. At the first meeting between family members and the home care nurse, family members expressed concern about their ability to do the intermittent catheterization procedure (ICP). The patient was worried about her bladder condition because she had heard that some patients had permanent bladder problems after hysterectomy.

After the first meeting, the nursing assessment was made and the following problems identified: (a) family and patient anxiety related to lack of knowledge of the ICP procedure after discharge; (b) urinary retention related to environmental and emotional stress, and weakened abdominal muscle; and (c) constipation related to stress and inadequate fluid intake. The patient and caregiver were educated about the normal recovery process of bladder function and were shown several techniques to stimulate urination. The patient was encouraged to void every 4 hours and to observe for signs of infection including checking her temperature. Also, the home care nurse showed the daughter-in-law how to sterilize equipment in boiling water and do the catheterization, and had her perform a return demonstration. She also gave them information about where they could buy supplies for ICP.

The first home visit was made on day 1 after discharge. The home care nurse found that all supplies were purchased and had been sterilized as instructed. ICP was done by the home care nurse and urinary retention was measured as 100 mL, and then the daughter-in-law was asked to perform the same procedure. She proceeded to demonstrate that she was a great student. She performed all of the procedures correctly, but she asked that the home care nurse would visit a few more times for support. Regarding her constipation after the operation, the patient could not have a bowel movement (BM) without an enema, and the amount was small. The patient complained about pain during the BM and lack of ability to push down strongly. Hard stool was palpated at the right lower quadrant. The patient was taught how to do abdominal massage, taught abdominal breathing to strengthen the abdominal muscle, and encouraged to consume a high-fiber diet and at least 2,000 mL of water per day. During a demonstration of abdominal massage and abdominal breathing, the patient went to the rest room and reported that she had a large satisfactory BM.

On day 2 and 3 postdischarge, the second and third home visits were made. The patient still complained about frequent urination, every 2 to 3 hours, with 30 to 120 mL of residual urine. Residual urine was checked twice a day. Because the amount of urine retention was stabilized, the daughter-in-law was informed that a urinary retention (UR) check-up was not necessary if it was maintained at less than 75 mL. The patient had a daily BM.

On day 6 after discharge, the last visit was made. ICP was done twice a day, and UR was 20 to 70 mL. The urine was a clear straw color and no sediment was noticed. Temperature and blood pressure were normal. The patient had small BMs 3 times a day. Therefore, ICP was discontinued, and the patient was discharged from home care services. On day 9 after discharge, the patient was followed by telephone and reported that she had regained normal urination and BM without pain, and she had visited a neighbor.

Case 2

A 67-year-old married man had experienced a cerebral vascular accident. He had left-sided weakness 8 months earlier but recovered in 2 weeks without intervention. The patient was brought to the emergency department in a confused mental state, with right-sided weakness and has been diagnosed with brain infarction. After 94 days in the hospital, the patient's condition had not been improved despite interventions; therefore, the family asked to take the patient home. The patient was referred to a home care nurse for home care services. He was stuporous, quadriplegic, and receiving gastric-tube feeding, on a tracheostomy with a Koken tube number 10. He had skin lesions on the left iliac crest and two open wounds on the right iliac crest, 2 x 1 cm. In addition, the patient had a history of hypertension and diabetes mellitus type II controlled with oral diabinase. Before the attack, the patient checked his blood sugar level and administered medicine by himself; therefore, the patient's wife did not know how to measure and administer the medicine.

This patient had two sons and three daughters, and lived with his two unmarried working daughters and his wife. During the hospitalization, the unmarried second daughter took a leave of absence from work to take care of him, but when he was discharged, she planned to go back to work. Therefore, when the patient was discharged, the wife was going to be the primary caregiver. Although the married daughter and first son lived in a distant province, they would visit every week, and the second son who lived close by would visit every day. In addition, the two sons took all financial responsibility including health care fees and monthly expenses. In accordance with the wishes of the family, plans to care for the patient at home and to allow the patient to die in the comfort of his own home were respected. The patient was discharged on day 103 after admission, with the gastric tube and tracheostomy.

The family had several strengths to draw on in developing a plan of care. An intact family system with open lines of communication facilitated planning. After meeting with the patient's family and reviewing the medical record, nursing assessments were made as follows: (a) family anxiety related to lack of knowledge about caring for the patient at home, (b) impaired skin condition related to immobility, (c) gastric-tube feedings and site care, (d) tracheostomy care and suctioning, and (e) risk of accident. A discharge care plan was made with family members, and the care plan and procedures were explained to them to reduce their anxiety and lack of confidence in performing the informal caregiver's role.

The list of supplies needed for home care was given to the family. Broad training was given to the family by the home care nurse. However, it was imperative that the family, especially the wife, gain a working knowledge of how to manage the gastric-tube feeding and tracheostomy suction. At least one family member had stayed with the patient in the hospital around the clock for more than 100 days, and they had learned suctioning and tube feeding from the nurses and practiced while they stayed with the patient.

The first home visit was 2 days after discharge. The patient's wife expressed her anxiety and stated, "I am really nervous, and I palpitate whenever he coughs." The home care nurse demonstrated suction and asked the wife to perform the suctioning and reassured her that her suctioning skills were excellent. For tracheostomy and gastric-tube feeding care, the nurse taught the wife how to monitor for signs and symptoms of systemic and local infection, maintain aseptic technique for inner cannula cleansing and replacement, tracheostomy site and gastric-tube site care, and hand washing vigorously before any procedures. For skin problems, the home care nurse demonstrated dressing changes on the wound and taught the wife about the sites where most skin problems occurred and how to maintain skin integrity through frequent position changes and back massage. Also, the nurse observed that the family accurately managed discharge medications and tube feeding and encouraged the family to express their feelings and to call the nurse when they had problems in caring for the patient.

The patient and family managed well for 3 months. During that time, supervised and taught by the home care nurse, the wife managed the gastric-tube feedings and suctioning, and provided skin care and physical therapy. Ninety days after discharge from the hospital, a gradual physical and mental deterioration began with increasing general edema, a large amount of secretions from the tracheostomy, and multiple third-stage wounds on the buttocks. The patient's wife was concerned about the financial burden to her children and worried about her physical and mental condition because she was getting weaker and depressed. The thought of what the meaning of her husband's life was if he lived in a vegetative state made her give up taking care of him; consequently, she did not check his blood sugar or blood pressure.

On the 101st day after discharge, the wife found the patient dead when she came into the patient's room for tube feeding after spending an hour with a friend who visited her that morning.

DISCUSSION

What are the future directions of home care nursing in Korea?

Cases 1 and 2 are useful not because they are typical home care cases today, but because they illustrate emerging issues for informal caregivers in terms of physical, psychological, and financial burden as well as issues of education and collaborative interdisciplinary work among health care professionals and paraprofessionals for home care nursing in Korea. Many problems in home care settings can be predicted and, therefore, effectively managed.

Providing home care for a sick family member is clearly a great burden and produces excessive stress (Kim, 1992). The evidence indicates that family members reach a point where they are overwhelmed by the burden and stress from uncertainty; lack of systematic education about assessment and the patient's prognosis; and absence of available systematic support, such as insurance-paid nurse aids. Therefore, in the second case described previously, the primary caregiver reached a point where she could no longer provide the care needed by her older husband.

This factor of family burden, preference, and demand for technological and financial support will be a restraining force of unknown magnitude in home care nursing and health care in general in Korea. These case studies suggest that nurses are beginning to develop a profile of the family that is capable of using technology to enhance patient care, but nothing has appeared in the literature yet to assist clinical decision making about high acuity and terminally ill patients' care in home settings.

The informal caregiver's motivation and confidence in learning and performing complicated technology for sick patients will be a major factor in determining the limits of success of home care nursing. Home care nurses should be more involved not only in assessment and education of informal caregivers, but also in direct patient care rather than depending primarily on informal caregivers. They should consult with other departments, use nurse aides to reduce the burden on informal caregivers, and work with financial departments on paying the cost of hiring nurse aides by insurance.

Support from other departments is lacking in home care and in acute care settings in Korea because of lack of specialization in physical, occupational, and recreation therapy, and medical social work. This means that nurses may have to cover all the home care client's health problems and also play the role of social worker. Moreover, one of the most problematic issues in home care nursing is supplies and equipment; there are few home care equipment suppliers, and most companies are linked with hospitals. Therefore, the individual patient or family must shop around. In these two cases, the family was given the list of supplies and stores rather than using vendors for home care.

Case 1 was a typical Korean patient with gastrourinary problems as a complication after abdominal surgery. Korean people tend to attribute an extremely wide range of complaints to the liver and gastrourinary tract including painful menstruation, and skin problems, such as acne, paleness, rash, and general fatigue (Lee, 1991, 1994). Embodied experiences are all the ways in which an individual conceptualizes and experiences his or her body (Kesselring, 1990). Body image is shaped by the social context in which these individuals are raised since this determines how to perceive and interpret the many body changes that occur over time in our own bodies. Death has been a mysterious and unsolvable riddle in the universe from prehistoric times. We can observe the viewpoints about death in every culture through the funeral rites and expressions of their ideas about the world after death. The influence of philosophy, culture, and morality on terminal home care nursing practice has to be considered while respecting each family's perception of death. Exposure in the classroom to ethical principles and rules will enable future nurses to examine the issues of critical or terminal care nursing, and the competing pressures in which they and their clients find themselves.

Finally, other factors may be considered in using home care including financial problems. Although health insurance pays in-hospital costs, it does not pay home care costs.

Home care administrators, government regulators, and the insurance industry should work closely together to create a better health care delivery system, using the benefits of home care nursing while reducing the physical, psychological, and financial burdens for the patient and family.

Overall, our perspective of the future for home care nursing is optimistic. We see a potential for growth that is capable of providing high-quality and culturally sensitive care to increasing numbers of patients, especially terminally ill or elderly patients. However, the partnership between informal caregiver and formal caregiver and interdisciplinary collaboration will be a major factor in determining the success of home care nursing in Korea.

REFERENCES

Kesselring, A. (1990). *The experienced body, when taken-for-grantedness falters: A phenomenological study of living with breast cancer.* Doctoral dissertation, University of California, San Francisco.

Kim, H. K. (1994). *The burden and health status of Informal caregivers to elderly patients.* Master's thesis, Yonsei University, Seoul, Korea.

Kim, S. S. (1992). *Experiences of family caregivers caring for the patients with stroke.* Doctoral dissertation, Yonsei University, Seoul, Korea.

Lee, H. O. (1991). Fatigue-transcultral issues in assessment and management. In H. P. Pritchard (Ed.), *European oncology nursing society* (pp. 138–140). Middlesex, England: Scutari.

Lee, H. O. (October 24, 1994). *Caring for the whole person: Blending therapies from around the world.* Paper presented at International AACN Conference, Toronto.

Lewin-VHI analysis of NAMES (National Association of Medical Equipment Suppliers) data. (1993). *The heavy burden of home care.* Washington, DC: Families USA.

Van Der Velde, C. D. (1985). Body image of one's self and of others: Developmental and clinical significance. *American Journal of Psychiatry, 142,* 527–537.

CHAPTER 14

Home-Based Psychiatric Services in Italy

Laura Cunico

CLOSURE OF PSYCHIATRIC HOSPITALS AND THE INTRODUCTION OF COMMUNITY-BASED PSYCHIATRIC SERVICES

In recent decades, various countries have experienced events that have brought about radical changes in the overall scene of psychiatric health care. One need think of only the Open Doors Movement in England, the Sector Psychiatry in France, and the community mental health centers in the United States. In Italy, change came about in psychiatric hospitals in the mid-1960s and is reflected in the studies carried out by Basaglia and his collaborators (Basaglia, 1968, 1981; Basaglia & Ongaro Basaglia, 1975). Basaglia's initial insights, which led to the founding of the *Movimento di Psichiatria Democratica* and whose ideas were supported by the "progressive" parties and public opinion in general, contributed to the passing of the law reform (Number 180) in 1978 (Siani, Siciliani & Burti, 1990). The most significant changes introduced by the new law were the following: (a) the hospitalization of a mentally disturbed person in a psychiatric hospital was no longer compulsory; (b) the introduction of diagnostic psychiatric services and treatment facilities in general hospitals (in cases of voluntary or compulsory hospitalization); (c) greater authority and responsibility were given to community-based health facilities located throughout the territory to provide basic psychiatric services; and (d) compulsory hospital treatment was restricted to limited cases. Voluntary treatment, the closure of psychiatric hospitals, and the decentralization of health services were the factors that inspired the new law.

Similarly, one can also imagine what sort of disruptive effect the new law had on the general hospital, which became the only facility available for psychiatric care and assistance. The physical space of the insane asylum, an enclosed, isolated environment, in which the most disparate needs were concentrated and left unattended, was now displaced in a short lapse of time by a variegated and complex system of community-based mental health services (Drigo, Borzaga, Mercurio & Satta, 1993).

PSYCHIATRIC CARE AND ASSISTANCE FACILITIES

The physical spaces where mental health care is now carried out are based in the community. These areas can be classified as *formal areas* (which include places where all the health services are provided, such as the local health authorities, the outpatient departments, the general hospital, etc.) and the *informal areas* (which are the places where patients normally live). Thus, the psychiatric care can, on the one hand, carry out its own specific function and, on the other, be integrated along with all the other health services into a general departmental health organization.

Psychiatric care includes a center for mental health, which represents the focal point of psychiatric services and the related activities of the psychiatric personnel (psychiatrists, psychologists, nurses, and social assistants). The psychiatric staff members are divided into multidisciplinary teams that attend to the overall needs of the patients either in the specific health facilities (exclusively or primarily in the case of mentally disturbed patients) or wherever a problem may arise requiring their presence (i.e., at the home or workplace).

People with emotional problems present different types of needs requiring personalized therapeutic programs; thus, a single-standard therapeutic procedure cannot be applied to all cases. The needs of each patient change over time and may occasionally require diversified services (i.e., treatment in outpatient departments, visits to the patient's home, temporary hospitalization, and rehabilitation therapies).

Two requirements emerge: on the one hand, there is a need to offer a *plurality of separate services,* each with its own specific function and, on the other hand, there is a need for some form of *coordination and integration* among them, so as to avoid wasteful overlapping or even gaps in the system.

Broadly speaking, the psychiatric services must, therefore, be organized in a such a way that they can be carried out in the various facilities of the Local Health Authorities and throughout the community. This includes both regularly planned operations and emergency operations, which presupposes a significant degree of mobility on the part of the psychiatric personnel. In addition, the health service must use *housing or semihousing facilities* with different degrees of security standards to accommodate and carry out rehabilitative therapies in cases where patients have serious psychological disturbances, a low level of autonomy, and problematic family situations.

The current scene in the Italian health care system indicates that the network of services, which involves specialized personnel, has not always been put into effect as the new law had intended. Consequently, we can observe a vast heterogeneity of situations from region to region, and from one Local Health Authority to another. However, in places where the reforms have actually been put into practice, that is, where psychiatric services concerning *psychiatric community services,* and *diagnosis* and *treatment* have been properly organized, the law reform has been a success. In fact, the reform has been applied in most areas of the country (Centro Studi Investimenti Sociali, 1985; Mosher & Burti, 1989; Tansella, De Salvia, & Williams, 1987).

MULTIDISCIPLINARY PSYCHIATRIC TEAMS AND THERAPEUTIC CONTINUITY

Operations concerning community-based psychiatric services are usually closely tied to an "organizational" work plan of community psychiatric teams. Each team is made up of different specialists, which includes psychiatrists with a support staff of psychologists, nurses, and social workers. Each member carries out a specific set of tasks; however, in the psychiatric setting, the role and function of each staff member are more elastic with respect to other sectors of the health service.

The homogenous and coherent make up of a multidisciplinary team does not however imply an overlapping of roles or relegating therapeutic responsibilities indiscriminately to all its members, which would lead to competitiveness and rivalry within the group. The group pools the specific skills and knowledge acquired from the day-to-day work experiences of each staff member (by use of work-study methods and special tools), so that each member can give his or her own particular contribution in creating the psychiatric team's specific therapeutic setting.

The team discusses each case and is responsible for planning the therapeutic objectives in assisting each individual patient. It is, therefore, necessary to circulate among all the staff members any information or assessments concerning the work carried out, the operative dynamics within the group, and any opposing views within the team itself (Siani et al., 1990).

Inevitably, every problematic case or new situation can lead to a divergence in opinions or a conflict of ideas within the work group; this is an innate feature of institutional dynamics. It is, therefore, inevitable that a therapeutic line will be constantly reexamined, clarified, and modified so as to ensure the collaboration of any staff members who may not fully agree with a certain line of approach to a particular problem (Siani et al., 1990).

One of the fundamental objectives in the community-based health system is that of *taking overall responsibility* for the patient. To do so, the staff of specialists must necessarily identify all the patient's needs and classify them; consequently, the team cannot maintain a rigid or preconceived organizational approach to each case. The way in which each team of specialists organizes itself will be defined according to the type of problem it is facing. Even the objective it aims to achieve is constantly reexamined and may change as a particular situation evolves.

At this point, the team's organizational problem becomes that of finding a point of equilibrium between a certain flexibility among staff members, which implies constantly constructing new approaches from one case to the next, and maintaining a planning function, which is necessary to ensure that the work is carried out in a systematic, coherent, and rational manner.

FUNCTION OF THE HOME CARE VISIT IN THE OVERALL SCHEME OF COMMUNITY-BASED SERVICES

The health care services provided at the patient's home are evaluated and coordinated at the local mental health center. The home care visit represents an important moment of contact with the patient's living environment. When a member of the medical staff (i.e., nurse or psychiatrist) crosses the threshold of the patient's home, he or she leaves behind the institutional arena and begins to share the suffering of those people who are close to the patient.

By bringing psychiatric services to the community, the field of vision is broadened from the single patient to the living environment of which the patient is an integral part. The psychiatric staff can now focus in on the network of relationships surrounding the patient and enter this network with a staff member acting as an active observer.

Thus, a staff member must leave the institutional confines and enter the patient's environment to understand both the patient and the group to which the patient belongs. A thorough understanding of the social setting in which the patient lives enables the staff member to make sense of the patient's mental disturbance, trace its history, and identify positive resources—such as the family, the neighbors, and the workplace—that might make an effective contribution to the therapeutic process. Friends, relatives, and acquaintances become a valid part of a therapeutic unit, allowing the patient to maintain interpersonal relations and carry out a specific role in society. This means acknowledging that the patient, who traditionally had been seen in only a rarefied and timeless atmosphere of a psychiatric hospital, is an individual with his or her own personal story.

Seen from this viewpoint, the home care visit can be considered, in the widest sense, a truly therapeutic act that occurs at different intervals of the patient's life.

USES OF HOME CARE VISITS

So far we have spoken about the home care visit as an important mode of intervening, and it is at times uniquely effective as a therapeutic activity in community-based health care. Now we shall look at the actual uses of the home care visit as a means of psychiatric care and assistance.

It is necessary to distinguish between the type of home care visit carried out in an emergency situation, which is in response to a "crisis," and those that are done in nonemergency conditions, which are a part of a planned series of activities decided on in advance by the visiting staff member (Siani et al., 1990).

In the first case, we need to consider several elements that are not strictly clinical, such as the type of request and its source—that is, who is making the request and in what context. In most cases, a staff member (often a nurse) at the mental health center is contacted by telephone by one of the members of the family. In other cases, and much less frequently, the person making the request is a general practitioner or a district health officer. However, the patient is rarely aware of the request being made on his or her behalf. This requires that the psychiatric team responds to family requests in an organized manner that will avoid any manipulative actions on the part of family members who solicit a visit from a staff member without informing the patient.

If hospitalization can be avoided, then home-based care can serve as a sort of *home hospitalization* where the patient is administered medicine, and a staff member can make daily and extended visits until the patient's crisis is under control.

In the second case, the home care visits are a part of a series of medical interventions planned in advance with the purpose of assisting the patient in the strictest sense of the term, especially in those cases in which the patient has undergone a prolonged stay in the hospital and requires readjusting socially to an external environment. Accordingly, the patient is accompanied and advised by a nurse in carrying out administrative tasks, searching for a home, paying utilities, organizing domestic chores, and so on. In addition, the home visit becomes particularly important when it is done for rehabilitative purposes, such as in the case of chronically psychotic patients who require support because of an inability to adapt and function to normal daily activities. From this viewpoint, the rehabilitative visit is based on the principle of stimulating patients to initiate activities and reacquire their personal skills to rediscover themselves as individuals and their roles in society.

BRIEF SURVEY OF HOME-BASED
CARE IN ITALY

The situation in Italy concerning home-based care has been influenced by the French-sector model since the 1960s. In Northern Italy, the home visit was initially used with the idea of preventing hospitalization in cases where patients had been released from psychiatric hospitals. Later, the experience of deinstitutionalizing and closing psychiatric hospitals in Gorizia, Arezzo, and Trieste further extended the use of home-based care so that it now assumed the overall responsibility of the needs of the patient within the family setting and in the community.

It is worth noting that the development of the home-based care also meant upgrading the professional qualifications of certain health personnel, especially in the case of nurses who, having left the psychiatric hospital and abandoned the role of a custodian, became an integral part of the change in the system.

The first work (Contini, 1978) describes the inception and evolution of home-based care concerning the *Ospedale Psichiatrico Cerletti di Parabiago*. The home visits were initially carried out by the social assistant with the purpose of ascertaining the real economic and housing conditions of the families of patients who were to be released from the hospital, and eventually helping these families cope with accepting the patient back into the family unit.

Subsequently, nurses began working together with social assistants on home visits and soon became the real protagonists in the community-based health service. Alongside the social assistant's duties during the home visit, the nurse assumed the responsibility of monitoring the patient and, in particular, checking the patient's behavior during his or her stay at home. Home-based care became part of a personalized therapeutic project and, as such, an integral part of outpatient services.

Bezoari (1980) identified three functions of the home-based care: a checking function, an understanding function, and a control function of the psychiatric team's internal operations. He also emphasized the risk the health staff faced in urgent situations, where the health officers are asked to maintain a delicate balance between two extremes of, on the one hand, leaving people in a crisis without any assistance and, on the other hand, mindlessly barging in on their lives and environment by way of "systematic interventions" (Petrella & Bezoari, 1982).

Using the experiences of Parabiago, Lanzara (1985) highlighted the evolution of the home-based care from the viewpoint of the staff members' expectations; namely, it had initially been idealized but subsequently perceived as an obligation, which led to a net fall in the quality of the service. The staff members were forced to acknowledge the difficulty in relating to a patient on a dimension that was different from that of the institution, and that the patient, capable of a partial autonomy, can also refuse a staff member's visit and obstruct the course of a therapeutic program.

Lastrucci (1990) classified five types of home-based care: *health,* having to do with the clinical evaluation of the patient and the environmental context; *assistance,* centered on helping the patient adapt to a social and family life; *relational,* aimed at obtaining knowledge of the patient's personal, social, and family relationships; *rehabilitative,* helping the patient reacquire social skills; and *institutional,* primarily concerned with aspects of social control.

Pittini (1978) was the first to open the descriptive-epidemiological line of research of home-based care. Pittini described 3 months of activity of the *Settori dell'Ospedale Psichiatrico Cerletti di Parabiago.* Most of the home-based care interventions were done with schizophrenic patients, and in general the visits tended to be personalized.

Straticò (1982, 1984) carried out a study concerning four Local Health Authorities in the province of Mantua. The study involved patients mostly between ages 45 and 65, pensioners, and people in a lower economic bracket with health assistance problems. The most frequent diagnosis was that of *functional psychosis* (55% of the cases) and *organic psychosis* (21%). The home visits were carried out mostly by nurses, alone or in pairs. In most cases the visits were concerned with the patient and fewer of the visits with the family members. The psychiatric interview was centered mainly on checking the clinical conditions of the patient. In most cases, once the visit was completed, the staff member discussed the results with the psychiatrist and, to a lesser extent, with the other staff nurses.

The book *Psichiatria a domicilio* (Cocchi, Contini, Berlincioni & Zanelli Quarantini, 1987), presented data regarding 6 months of home interventions carried out in 1986 at the *Centro Psicosociale di Magenta,* in Milan. The staff members followed cases of 60 home-based patients and carried out 480 home-based care interventions. However, the nurses' specific contribution in these home-based interventions does not emerge from the study. The most frequent diagnosis was that of schizophrenic psychosis. The patients were mainly female (57%) and represented mostly age groups 36 to 50 (50%) and 51 to 65 (27%), whereas, there was only a minimal presence of younger patients (15% younger than 35 years of age).

At the conference, The Psychiatric Visit at Home, held in Lucca, Lazzerini, Andreani, and Raimondi (1990) presented data related to home-based care interventions carried out in Massa Carrara (8,862 visits involving 202 patients). Fifty percent of the patients had been diagnosed with schizophrenic psychosis; 20%, manic-depression; 9%, neurosis; 9%, organic psychosis; and 6%, alcohol addiction.

During the same conference, Scatena, Cirillo, Martinelli, Rocca, and De Cesari (1990) presented data relating to home-based care carried out in 1988 in Garfagnana. These visits represented 27% of the overall inter-ventions of the health service.

The types of intervention were defined as follows: 56% were health; 27%, institutional; 6%, assistance; 6%, relational; and 5%, rehabilitative.

The interventions were done only by nurses in 78% of the cases; doc-tors together with nurses in 18% of the cases; and doctors and psycholo-gists in 4% of the cases. If we consider the patients, the nurses operated alone in 57% of the cases, and a nurse together with a doctor in 39% of the cases.

The Labos study entitled *Utenza Psichiatrica e Servizi* (1986), funded by the Center of Studies of the Ministry of Health, surveyed home-based care interventions carried out in four regions (Piedmont, Umbria, Puglia, and Basilicata) during the period January–June 1985. The most frequent diagnosis was that of schizophrenia (62%), whereas other dis-orders to a lesser extent included affective disturbances (14%), neuro-sis (12%), personality disorders (6%), and organic psychosis (6%).

Home-based care visits were carried out especially in cases where patients were seriously ill; namely, schizophrenics, long-term outpa-tients, and patients with problematic family situations. According to the family members, the staff member who was most involved in this ser-vice was the nurse (represented by 57% of the responses given by fam-ily members); followed by the family doctor; and, to a lesser extent, the psychologist and the social assistant. The reasons cited most often included performing periodic checks of the patient's clinical condition (49%), administering medication (13%), and helping the patient with domestic chores and personal hygiene (11%). The main type of activity at the patient's home was psychiatric interviewing (81%), and administering prescription drugs and checking the psychological conditions of the patient, represented 39% of the activities. The study showed that the types of intervention that were done most widely were also consistent with what family members considered most useful, such as psychiatric interviewing, administering medication, and advising the family members. Nevertheless, the family members suggested that the number of interventions aimed at checking the patient's state of health and of a rehabilitative nature should be increased.

The home-based care interventions were most frequent in Umbria compared with those in Basilicata, and their main purpose was that of preventing crises. In addition, the psychiatric interview, checking the patient's state of health, and providing support and advice to family members were also more frequent in Umbria compared with the other regions. The psychiatrist was the staff member most involved in home-based care in Puglia and Basilicata, whereas, the nurse intervened most frequently in Umbria and Piedmont.

A multicenter study was done on nine *Centri Psicosociali* in Lombardy by Lora et al. (1995), which tried to define the process of home-based care. The results showed that interventions of this kind were directed primarily toward female patients between the ages of 45 and 65, diagnosed with psychosis, unmarried, and long-term patients of the home-based treatment program. The psychiatric staff member who had actually carried out the home-based care was a nurse in 9 cases out of 10 (a nurse was present alone in 69% of the cases; two nurses, 23%; a social assistant, 9%; a doctor, 7%; a psychologist, 0.5%; and an education official, 1%).

The contact time with the patient during the intervention was on average 25 minutes. The main objective of the home-based care treatment in 8 cases out of 10 seemed to be that of evaluating and checking the patient's psychiatric conditions (81%); other objectives included evaluating the family relationships (30%); administering therapeutic medication (32%); and providing emotional support and reassuring the patients (34%). Still other objectives, though less frequent included giving emotional support to family members (21%), evaluating the patient's physical health (13%), and helping the patient with personal hygiene (19%). The topics that were dealt with most frequently during the interview were the psychiatric symptoms of the patient (47%), the patient's relationship with the people he or she was living with (34%), and issues arising from day-to-day life (38%). The less frequent subjects during the interview had to do with the patient's physical health (23%), personal hygiene (19%), and problems or difficulties reported by those living with the patient.

If we shift our attention from the psychiatric interview to some of the practical activities carried out by the staff member during the home visit, we can observe that in more than half the cases medication was administered to the patient. The home-based care remains above all closely tied with the psychiatric interview and the relationship between staff member and patient, in which practical activities do not have a primary function.

The home-based care does not end when the staff member leaves the patient. The information is reported back to and discussed with the other members of the psychiatric team, and, in particular, with the psychiatrist responsible for treating the patient.

The cluster analysis has enabled us to identify, at least in part, several typologies of home-based care. The first represents the type of psychiatric intervention relating to control and supervision, in which attention is given primarily to the interview between staff member and patient concerning problems of a psychiatric and relational nature. In the second type, the psychiatric aspect becomes more "interventionist"; that is, the nurse administers medication and focuses the psychiatric interview on problems of a psychiatric nature. The third type is rehabilitative and resocializing in the sense that the activities are finalized in caring for the patient, the home setting, and reintroducing the patient to recreational activities; consequently, the psychiatric interview does not touch on any psychiatric issues. Besides these profiles of home-based care, there is also a fourth mixed group that integrates all the various aspects of intervention; it is from this group that the visiting staff member derives a subjective feeling of being more useful and, thus, derives greater professional satisfaction.

In addition, researchers are discussing the possibility of expanding the scope of home-based care by integrating psychoeducational techniques into the home-based activities.

A recent study (Burti & Tansella, 1995) reports the home visit of the community-based psychiatric service of South Verona in the period 1982 to 1991. The study highlights a pattern that has developed over the years concerning the length of stay in a hospital and home visits. There has been a progressive decrease in the number of days the patient remains in the hospital and a corresponding increase in the number of home care visits. The mean number of occupied beds per day (ratio per 10,000) was 4.8 in 1991, that is, 28.6% lower than in the 1982 ratio (6.7 per 10,000) and 48.8% lower than the 1979 ratio (9.3 per 10,000). Conversely, the number of home visits provided in 1991 ($n = 1,824$) was 786% higher than in 1982 ($n = 232$) and in 1979 ($n = 233$).

Three diagnostic groups were considered: (a) schizophrenia and relative disorders; (b) affective disorders; and (c) all other diagnoses. Over this period, women between 45 and 65 years of age, suffering from schizophrenia and relative and affective disorders, received the greatest number of home care visits compared with younger women and men (< 45 years).

The authors point out that although there had been an increase in the number of home visits, there had also been a parallel increase in alternative forms of assistance offered by the health service, such as day care, outpatient care, and rehabilitation programs.

However, the authors asserted that before coming to the conclusion that the decrease in hospital care is correlated to the increasing provision of psychiatric and psychological services in patient home care programs, more studies and analysis of case-register data are required.

CONCLUSIONS

By shifting the focal point of health care from the hospital to the community, psychiatric reform in Italy has favored the gradual evolution of duties of psychiatric nurses, that is, from a function primarily consisting of *control* and *custody* to a function of providing *health care* and *assistance.*

The brief survey of studies presented in this chapter clearly shows the central role of the nurse in home-based care as concerns the field of community-based psychiatric services. The main tasks that characterize the nurse's role include maintaining a therapeutic relationship with the patient and members of the family, monitoring and treating the patient's psychotic symptoms, and evaluating the patient's ability to cope with daily life.

It is important for the nurse who is carrying out a home-based intervention to know who the patient is, what the planned activities are, and what the objective of the intervention is. Home-based care has to be organized both within the psychiatric team at the mental health center and with the patient and family members because the home setting often tends to distort the objectives of the intervention and sometimes even the role of the nurse.

The visiting staff member and patient relationship runs a risk of becoming chronic over time, even though the particular patient's case is discussed and reexamined within the team, thus motivating the members of the team to search for alternative approaches.

Thus, the nurse is the main figure in this type of health service and is responsible for carrying out this role with a therapeutic purpose. This can only be achieved if there is a clear therapeutic program shared by the entire psychiatric team, the patient, and the family members.

A still-unexplored area of the psychiatric nursing in Italy concerns *psychoeducation*. This technique could be integrated with home-based care as was suggested by the authors of the study done in Lombardy.

The psychoeducational approach, in its various and different techniques, as proposed by Anderson, Reiss, and Hogarty (1986), Faloon et al. (1982, 1985), Leff (1987), Tarrier (1988), and Tarrier et al. (1989), and consistent with the historical prerequisites of research on expressed emotion (Brown, Birley & Wing, 1972), is aimed at reducing the risks of a relapse in the case of a schizophrenic patient.

The main approaches in achieving this objective are (a) informing the family members on the nature of the disease of a schizophrenic patient; (b) adjusting their expectations; (c) establishing an alliance with the family to ensure its cooperation until the patient is on regular therapeutic medication (pharmatherapeutic compliance); and (d) training members of the family and correcting their emotional responses to the psychotic symptoms and behavior of the patient.

These topics receive a great deal of attention in home-based care, but have rarely been the subjects of a detailed study. They are also neglected too often, even though adequate information is constantly requested by family members, as pointed out by Kuipers (1992). For example, it is well known that the family environment can influence the symptoms of a schizophrenic patient, just as it is also well known that family members have to bear a great emotional burden living with a psychotic patient (Fadden, Bebbington, & Kuipers, 1987).

Oftentimes, no adequate explanation concerning schizophrenia is given to the family, whereas most of the attention is given to relational aspects within the home-based care.

The psychoeducational approach could prove to be a useful operative method in home-based care. The planning of the overall treatment program and the timing of specific interventions within the home setting enables the nurse to better meet the needs of the patients and those of the family members.

REFERENCES

Anderson, C. M., Reiss, D. J., & Hogarty, G. E. (1986). *Schizophrenia and family: A practitioner's guide to psychoeducation and management.* New York: Guilford.

Basaglia, F. (1968). *Le istituzioni della violenza.* In F. Basaglia (Ed.), *L'istituzione negata.* Torino, Italy: Einaudi.

Basaglia, F. (1981). *Opere.* Torino, Italy: Einaudi.

Basaglia, F., & Ongaro Basaglia, F. (Eds.) (1975). *Crimini di pace.* Torino, Italy: Einaudi.

Bezoari, M., Gesué, A., & Fiamminghi, A. M. (1980). La visita domiciliare in psichiatria: Considerazioni metodologiche. *Quadrangolo, 33,* 12–14.

Brown, G. W., Birley, J. L. T., & Wing, J. K. (1972). Influence of family life on the course of schizophrenic disorders: A replication. *British Journal of Psychiatry, 121,* 241–258.

Burti, L., & Tansella, M. (1995). Acute home-based care and community psychiatry. In M. Phelan, G. Strathdee, & G. Thornicroft (Eds.), *Emergency in mental health services in the community.* Cambridge, England: Cambridge University Press.

Centro Studi Investimenti Sociali. (1985). *L'attuazione della riforma psichiatrica ne quadro delle politiche regionali e dell'offerta quantitativa e qualitativa dei Servizi.* (Rapporto conclusivo di indagine sul censimento e analisi dei servizi psichiatrici). Roma, Italy: Author.

Cocchi, A., Contini, A., Berlincioni, V., & Zanelli Quarantini, F. (1987). *Psichistria a domicilio.* Milano, Italy: Franco Angeli Editore.

Contini, A. (1978). Evoluzione dell'attività domiciliare. In D. De Martis & M. Bezoari (Eds.), *Istituzione, famiglia, Equipe curante.* Milano, Italy: Feltrinelli.

Contini, A. (1987). Il processo di trasformazione dell'intervento domiciliare nell'evoluzione di un centro psichiatrico territoriale: Una lettura sistemica. In A. Cocchi et al. (Eds.), *Psichiatria a domicilio.* Milano, Italy: Franco Angeli Editore.

Drigo, M. L., Borzaga, L., Mercurio, A., & Satta, E. (1993). *Clinica e Nursing in Psichiatria.* Milano, Italy: Casa Editrice Ambrosiana.

Fadden, G., Bebbington, P., & Kuipers L. (1987). The burden of care. *British Journal of Psychiatry, 150,* 285.

Fallon, I. R. H., Boyd, J. L., McGill, C. W., Razani, J., Moss, H. B., & Gilderman, A. M. (1982). Family management in the prevention of exacerbations of Schizophrenia. *New England Journal of Medicine, 306,* 1437–1440.

Faloon, I. R. H., Boyd, J. L., McGill, C. W., Williamson, M., Razani, J., Moss, H. B., Gilderman, A. M., & Simpson, G. M. (1985). Family management in the prevention of morbidity of schizophrenia: Clinical outcome of a two-years longitudinal study. *Archives of General Psychiatry, 42,* 887–896.

Kuipers, L. (1992). Needs of relatives of long-term psychiatric patient. In G. Thornicroft, C. Brewin, & J. Wing. (Eds.), *Measuring mental health needs.* (p. 291). London: Gaskell.

LABOS (Laboratorio per le politiche sociali) (1986). *Utenza psichiatrica e servizi: Ricerca promossa dal Centro Studi del Ministero della Sanità.* Roma, Italy: Edizioni TER.

Lanzara, D. (1985). Le visite domiciliari. In M. Tognetti Bordogna (a cura di) (Ed.), *I muri cadono adagio: Storia dell'ospedale psichiatrico di Parabiago.* Milano, Italy: Franco Angeli Editore.

Lastrucci, P. (1990). Introduzione al tema al tema del convegno. *Fogli di informazione, 146,* 13–16.

Lazzerini, F., Andreani, M. F., & Raimondi R. (1990). Il registro dei casi psichiatrici come strumento di rilevazione della visita a domicilio del paziente. *Fogli di informazione, 146,* 121–125.

Leff, J. P. (1987). Two trials of intervention in families of schizophrenic patients: Theoretical and practical implications (Relazione al Workshop internazionale "Shizofrenia e Famiglia: Modelli a Confronto," Milano, 1–3 luglio 1987, trad.it. Due fasi di intervento in famiglie di pazienti schizofrenici: implicazioni teoriche e pratiche). *Notizie ARS, 2,* (Suppl. 3), 30–40.

Lora, A., Bellini, S., Bertoli, A., Bezzi, R., Cassis, I., Comelli, M., Gandini, A., Magnani, G., Migliaretti, G., Paganesi, M., Percudani, M., Pezzullo, M., & Morosini, P. (1995a). Aspetti valutativi dell'intervento domiciliare in psichiatria: 1. *Rivista Sperimentale di Freniatria, 119,* 29–53.

Mosher, L. R., & Burti, L. (1989). *Community mental health: Principles and practice.* New York: Norton.

Petrella, F., & Bezoari, M. (1982). Lo psichiatra a casa del paziente: Una nuova area operativa e conoscitiva. In M. Lang (a cura di) (Ed.), *Strutture intermedie in psichiatria.* Milano, Italy: Raffaele Cortina Editore.

Pittini, G. (1978). Esposizione e commento dei dati quantitativi. In D. De Martis & M. Bezoari (a cura di) (Eds.), *Istituzione, famiglia, Equipe curante.* Milano, Italy: Feltrinelli.

Scatena, P. A., Cirillo, M., Martinelli, M., Rocca, R., & De Cesari, A. (1990).

A domicilio del paziente psichiatrico: 1. Gli interventi programmati. *Fogli di informazione, 146,* 39–45.

Siani, R., Siciliani, O., & Burti, L. (1990). *Strategie di Psicoterapia e Riabilitazione.* Milano, Italy: Feltrinelli Editore.

Straticò, E. (1982). *La visita domiciliare psichiatrica: Ostiglia, Italy: USSL 48.* (USSL n. 48 della). Ostiglia: Lombardia.

Straticò, E. (1984). La visita domiciliare in psichiatria. *Prospettive sociali e sanitarie, 20,* 7.

Tansella, M., De Salvia, D., & Williams, P. (1987). The Italian psychiatric reform: Some quantitative evidence. *Social Psychiatric, 22,* 37–48.

Tarrier, N. (1988, September 22). The family management of schizophrenia within a community setting. Paper presented to the "Course in Community Psychiatry," Institute of Psychiatric Demography, Aarhus, Denmark.

Tarrier, N., Barrowclough, C., Vaughn, C., Bamrah, J. S., Porceddu, K., Watts, S., & Freeman H. L. (1989). Community management of schizophrenia: A two years follow-up of a behavioral intervention with families. *British Journal of Psychiatry, 154,* 625–628.

CHAPTER 15

Psychiatric Home Care Nursing in the United States

Katherine Jubell Proehl and Rose Anne M. Berila

Psychiatric home care is an important component in the management of the mentally ill. It provides quality care in a cost-effective manner when done well. Home care is most often initiated when the client is either in or near crisis, or has just been through a hospitalization and is not yet able to care for himself or herself fully. The nurse's goal is to assist the client in the stabilization process and help prevent relapses. Her or his work is individualized because of the clients' varied needs. Often clients have been frequent users of health care resources: excessive telephone calls from the client or family members to the primary psychiatric clinician, recurrent visits to the emergency room, and multiple psychiatric admissions to the hospital are common. These clients have needs that are not being met by more traditional health care services. Having the nurse care for the clients in their own home is the least restrictive means of treatment and allows the caregiver to individualize care to best meet the client's needs.

The psychiatric home care nurse will generally follow two types of patient populations. The first consists of patients with chronic mental illnesses who do not have the support or guidance they need to achieve their optimal level of functioning. Relapse and medication noncompliance are frequent problems that psychiatric home care can minimize. The second group of patients has acute episodes of mental illness. These patients are generally followed by the nurse for a limited time to assist them in moving through their psychiatric crisis. Examples are patients experiencing severe major depressive episodes or an exacerbation of an anxiety disorder. Care of clients with severe personality disorders requires time-limited, realistic goals that are focused and clearly understood by the client.

Reimbursement requirements vary depending on the payer. Generally, there are three basic requirements. First, the patient must have a psychiatric diagnosis. Second, the client must be "homebound." Psychiatric homebound status generally means the patient is unable to access psychiatric follow-up independently and consistently. This is a wide definition that is interpreted differently in varying geographic regions. The last requirement is that the client must require the skills of a psychiatric nurse.

This chapter describes the nature of psychiatric home care nursing. Information provided in the ensuing case histories is based on firsthand experience in this field. Each case is followed by a brief discussion. The cases are typical of the population followed.

CASE STUDIES

Case 1

An 84-year-old married man was diagnosed with dementia, chronic obstructive pulmonary disease, hypertension, coronary artery disease, and asthma; depression was ruled out. Psychiatric home care was ordered for him on discharge from an inpatient psychiatric unit. The question of whether this patient needed to be placed in a nursing home was a concern of the treatment team. Before his hospitalization, his family was having great difficulty managing him at home. His confusion had become significantly worse, and he was increasingly agitated to the point that he hit his aged wife over the head with his cane. While hospitalized, it was discovered that the client was clearly overmedicated, and this was contributing to his confused mental status. His medicines were adjusted, and he was sent home after a brief hospitalization.

I had the chance to briefly meet this patient in the hospital and spoke to his wife on the telephone before our first visit. The patient's wife was relieved to have help. The client initially was resistant to my visits, denying the need for help of any kind. He was a man with great pride and had difficulty accepting his declining mental status. This made safety a difficult issue for his family. This man lived with his wife in the two-story home in which they had raised their children. All the children lived in the area and were actively involved with caring for their parents.

The client was having difficulty giving up control in his life. Despite his confusion, he would try and drive the car, or at times, he would sneak out of the house alone to take a walk and end up lost in a dangerous neighborhood. It was clear that the patient's wife dearly loved her husband, but because of his mental deficits in some areas, she had fallen into the pattern of attempting to control all aspects of her husband's life. This tended to frustrate the client, and fights frequently broke out that often became physical. The assessment of the patient and the immediate circumstances indicated that safety was a primary concern for the family.

Interventions were focused at several levels. First, I worked with the patient's wife on correctly dispensing her husband's medicine. Because of multiple medical problems, he was on an elaborate medication schedule that neither he or his wife understood or were able to follow. I contacted the patient's various doctors and helped his wife clarify dosages, times, and frequencies. Next, I assisted them in designing a pill box that they understood and could easily use. Over time, I also worked with his wife on appropriately using medicine as needed to help manage the patient's agitation in a safe manner.

My work with this patient was mostly focused on validating his strengths and listening to his life story. This simple intervention was calming for him. We focused on what he could remember, and I was careful not to frustrate him by dwelling on topics that confused him. Safety measures in the home were also addressed.

Helping the patient's wife learn to manage her husband without the situation escalating into a violent power struggle was an important intervention. I used role modeling and direct feedback in aiding her to deal with her husband—for example, helping her decide when to remain firm and when to acquiesce. The patient's wife learned that unless there was a safety concern, her husband should be allowed to have his way in matters concerning himself. This change clearly improved this man's mood and decreased most of the verbal fighting and all the physical battles.

The client progressed well in the home environment. Treatment was abruptly stopped because of his sudden death by cardiac arrest. When his wife called to tell me her husband had died, she emphasized how grateful the entire family was. Their worst fear was having to place this man in a nursing home. She was upset about his death but verbalized feeling good about being able to manage the last part of her husband's life in her home.

This situation illustrates the importance of working with the caregivers of the primary patient. In this case, most of my work revolved around teaching the family how best to help the patient. The quality of life for the client and his wife was clearly affected by having a psychiatric home care nurse.

Discussion

In case 1, the home care nurse was able to realize that the interventions to help the patient live successfully at home were rooted in helping the family deal more effectively with his dementia. In dementing illnesses, the anchor for people losing their memory is their family because only their family can help others to see them as a person in the context of their lives. This is why the interventions were directed at the family. The patient in case 1 relied on his family to advocate for his needs for self-respect, autonomy, and self-esteem.

Helping the family work through the feelings associated with taking some of the decision making away from the husband or father is difficult work. It requires family members to work through feelings that are stirred up by changing roles within a family. These transitions represent major losses, and families must be allowed to acknowledge these losses and to grieve them. It is only after this has occurred, that the nurse can help a family to preserve some autonomy for the person with dementia and narrow their focus to such issues as safety. The family eventually learned to give this patient control over some decisions to foster his self-esteem and autonomy without jeopardizing his safety. Without the home care nurse's skill in assisting this family in working through the losses mentioned, they would not have been able to narrow the focus to safety issues, the verbal and physical battles would have continued, and this patient might have needed placement.

Case 2

A 33-year-old married woman was diagnosed with a schizoaffective disorder. She had been hospitalized numerous times because of suicidal ideations and attempts to end her life. This woman had difficulty coping, especially when her auditory hallucinations would recur, telling her that she was evil and that she should kill herself. With each hospitalization, she felt more hopeless, and her fragile self-esteem plummeted. Psychiatric home care was ordered to increase her support and decrease the need for hospitalizations. She was groggy with a flat affect and was beginning to hear voices telling her to kill herself. After seeing this patient for several weeks, it became apparent that her medications needed adjustment. The patient's psychiatrist was notified and the frequency of home visits increased. This woman was resistant to the thought of returning to the hospital. Because the nurse's rapport with her was growing, she was able to contract for safety between visits. The decision was made to continue management of the patient in the home setting.

Safety was the first concern with this client. The initial plan required joining the husband and wife at her upcoming doctor's appointment. The psychiatrist was given a clear picture of what appeared to be going on with this woman at home. The decision of the minitreatment team, which included the client, her husband, the psychiatrist, and the nurse, was to change her long-standing neuroleptic medication. To monitor and support this client and her husband through this major change, I worked closely with the psychiatrist and saw this patient every day during her worst times. This woman's hallucinations initially worsened, and she became even more regressed. Her husband's hope was wearing down, but he was somewhat comforted by the close attention psychiatric home care brought to his wife. Monitoring response to medications and medication teaching were the major focus of my work with both the patient and her husband. I also spoke regularly with the doctor as we tapered her old medication and titrated up the new one. Eventually, all our hard work and attention began to pay off. The patient's thought process began to clear. Her hallucinations stopped, and her affect widened.

A pressing problem for this client was her withdrawn behavior, which historically contributed to her ineffective coping and eventual relapses. This client had difficulty performing activities of daily living (ADLs). These behaviors contributed to her feelings of low self-esteem and worthlessness. A cyclical pattern had developed in which this woman would allow her feelings to prevent her from taking better care of herself. The goal was to interrupt this cycle and assist the client in developing healthier behavioral patterns. A concrete behavioral plan was initiated, aiding the patient in structuring her day and affirming her strengths. The therapeutic relationship between the client and myself supported this woman in developing a new way of managing her feelings and behavior.

The psychiatric home care nurse develops a different relationship with clients than the caregiver who works in a more traditional setting. Therapeutic boundaries must be kept. Once the nurse walks into the client's home, a more intimate and personal relationship is bound to develop. The home care nurse becomes part friend, part family, part doctor, and part case manager, assisting the client in accessing appropriate health care resources. The home care nurse quickly gains a much greater understanding of the client's situation, and the client has more control than in a traditional setting. Even with therapeutic boundaries, the relationship that dévelops is more intimate.

Another significant part of the nursing care for this woman was assisting her in getting involved with activities outside her home. The patient had lost her job previously when her illness worsened. After several years of being isolated in her home, the client's confidence about doing simple tasks was shaky at best. She often would remark about desiring to return to work but was not sure she would be able to handle the pressure. She enrolled in a job-training program for the mentally ill, and with support from me, she interviewed and eventually was hired as a receptionist. Initially, this woman had difficulty mostly related to her poor interpersonal skills and at several points in time contemplated quitting. With support from her family and myself, however, she was able to work through the initial awkwardness on the new job and eventually found comfort in her work routine.

Around a year after my initial visit, the client stopped taking her medications and began stockpiling them. She was able to be honest about the noncompliance; this topic had been a regular part of our discussions. Unfortunately, several months later, I arrived at her home for our regularly scheduled visit to learn that the patient had taken an overdose of acetaminophen (Tylenol). I was aware that the patient had become more stressed because of recent family turmoil and that she felt powerless to stop the feuding. The client was hospitalized. Her overdose was calculated and clearly a cry for help. I believe it was related to her inability to assert her needs within her family and differed from previous attempts that were more related to her past psychotic states.

The patient was able to admit that she truly did not want to die but at that moment did not know what else to do. We discussed alternative ways of expressing despair and laid out a concrete suicide prevention plan in hopes of avoiding further life-threatening acts. Unfortunately, because of her thought disorder, the patient had difficulty understanding her behavior within her family system. In later sessions, we worked on exploring this dynamic within the family system with concrete terms and examples.

Since the last hospitalization this woman has done well. She returned to work and her mood appears brighter. Assertiveness training was added to the client's care plan, but she continues to struggle with this issue. Because of the chronic nature of her illness and her history of multiple hospitalizations before home care, this client was a good candidate for ongoing psychiatric home care.

Discussion

In case 2, the patient's chronicity and the family's inability to discuss and resolve family conflicts openly had to be respected by the home care nurse to gain acceptance and to build trust. In home care, the nurse is entering the patient's domain and must be respectful of the values, culture, and coping patterns found in the home, or the nurse will not be able to continue home visits. Although sensitivity to these issues is necessary in traditional outpatient therapy, the therapist has more control on his or her "turf" over how to confront issues. The risk of offending the patient does not necessarily result in the termination of visits. The down side of home care nursing can be having to tread more lightly when challenging the family system. This is balanced by the fact that being in the patient's home and seeing a family in its natural environment gives the nurse greater insights into the family's strengths as well as into the purpose the dysfunctional behavior serves.

The nurse in case 2 used an understanding of entering family systems in a home environment to maximize the patient and husband's strengths rather than confronting the resistance head on. This allowed the client to gain enough support from her family and self-confidence that she was able to return to work. Focusing on medication compliance and self-esteem allowed the patient and her family to grow and to slow the cycle of psychotic breaks. As a person or family system grows and changes, old coping mechanisms gradually become ineffective. When this woman could not verbalize her need for support during a time of significant family turmoil, she repeated the coping mechanism used in the past, she overdosed, but this time without regressing and becoming psychotic. This resulted in rehospitalization, getting the family to agree to some family therapy, and a resolution of the current family turmoil. As the patient and her family continue to grow, there will be the potential for learning healthier coping mechanisms and for developing more open communication during times of stress. This growth can only occur slowly over time. Psychiatric home care nurses must learn to respect the time table patients and families set for growth. Psychiatric home care nurses are also better able to help their clients if they are able to see what appear to be setbacks as faltering attempts at approximating healthier coping behaviors.

Case 3

A 74-year-old married woman had a severe reoccurrence of major depression. During her 30s, she had suffered her first bout with this illness but had not had a relapse of this magnitude since that time. She was not responding to outpatient therapy. Her psychiatrist was alarmed by the client's regressed state and had recommended inpatient electroconvulsive therapy (ECT) treatments. The client refused, voicing concerns about both the actual treatment and hospitalization. Psychiatric home care was ordered as a compromise in the hope that a different treatment modality might help.

On my first visit, this woman hesitantly let me in the house. She was disheveled, had poor eye contact, anxiously chain smoked, and was in the pajamas she had been wearing continuously for 3 days. Her affect was both sad and worried. She reported feeling exhausted despite not doing much aside from lying in bed. The content of her speech revolved around themes of guilt, helplessness, and hopelessness. She expressed a desire to be dead but would not kill herself because of her religious beliefs. She had made no attempts in the past. She had no children but was happily married for years. Her husband reported his wife's current behavior was uncharacteristic of her usual personality. She had lived an active life, only occasionally smoked, and had always been concerned about her appearance.

The home assessment was useful. It complemented the psychiatrist's assessment. The client appeared to be anxious on top of being depressed. This was something her doctor was unable to pick up in the office setting. Her anxiety greatly contributed to her discomfort and unwillingness to comply with previous treatment suggestions. In collaboration with her psychiatrist, her medication was adjusted, and a behavioral plan initiated. The plan included setting firmer limits on the patient's self-defeating behavior and medication to temporarily relieve anxiety while antidepressant medication was slowly increased.

The client was initially angry with me. Her husband no longer enabled her negative behavior and stopped taking responsibility for things the patient needed to be doing. The plan included being empathetic and acknowledging this woman's suffering. We focused on what was realistic for her to be doing at different times of her recovery. Realistic activities included dressing and bathing every day, going for her weekly appointment at the hair salon, letting close friends visit to offer support, and attempting to eat part of each meal seated with her husband at the kitchen table.

I also used supportive psychotherapy by allowing the client to vent feelings and thoughts, but set limits on how much I would listen to her negate and shame herself. The patient was initially so depressed that her thinking was often distorted. I gently helped her reframe unrealistic thoughts and reorient to reality. Medication and illness teaching for both the patient and her husband was important. Reinforcing the concept of depression as a treatable illness seemed to give this woman relief from her guilt and hopelessness. Helping the family understand the time frame in which antidepressant medications work also aided in building hope.

Initially, this patient was so depressed that she struggled to get to her doctor's appointments, let alone reach out to community resources. Because of home care, I was able to come to her on a regular basis and treat her in the least restrictive means possible. Hospitalization was avoided, and the patient was able to recover at home. This plan was both cost-effective and provided quality care.

The client's recovery was dramatic over the 2.5-month period I worked with her. Her anxiety lessened with the help of new relaxation techniques and medication. This allowed her to focus on the behavioral plan with success and gave her the patience to stay on her antidepressant medicine.

The discussed interventions are not unique to psychiatric nurses who work in home care. The home environment and the community are the "therapeutic milieu" in psychiatric nursing home care. The patient's home creates a different tone. Nursing care is more individualized and will more effectively involve the patient than therapy done in traditional settings. The home environment provides the nurse with a vast supply of information and means to creatively individualize care, while nurturing a special bond between the client and nurse. For example, the client's husband was able to identify numerous things his wife had always loved about her home and neighborhood. Her behavioral plan included activities that would place her in situations with the things she loved—hence, the environment positively supported goals and interventions.

Discussion

Case 3 illustrates the benefits of short-term home care in a patient's recovery from an acute episode of mental illness in a previously high-functioning person. Had the nurse not seen the patient in her home setting and gained access to the husband's insight and support, this woman could have continued to frustrate her outpatient therapist's attempts to help. From a cost-effectiveness standpoint, there is no doubt that 10 weeks of home visits is far less expensive than a week's hospitalization. From a patient perspective, mastering an episode of depression at home with the help of a nurse, psychiatrist, and family is far more empowering. This patient was allowed to participate more fully in her recovery than she could in a hospital. Having the client in her home also enhanced her relationship with her husband and his understanding about how to be supportive to his wife. The client's husband would not have been able to set limits and firmly encourage his wife to be more active without the home care nurse's support and role modeling.

Effective use of the home setting and the family as a therapeutic "milieu" is also well illustrated. The fact that the patient and her husband had many productive years together allowed the nurse to use their strengths in planning the patient's care. The client's husband had strengths different from those of the spouses in cases 1 and 2, and the nurse capitalized on these strengths for the benefit of the patient.

CONCLUSION

These three case histories illustrate an effective way psychiatric clients can be managed in the home. Several key points are evident. First, the home care nurse and psychiatrist must work closely together and be aligned in the treatment plan. Without the support of the psychiatrist, the nurse's effectiveness greatly decreases. Patients need to know that all their caregivers work together and are united. Nurses and psychiatrists must be receptive to each others' opinions and place the client's well-being first.

The therapeutic relationship developed between the client and the psychiatric home care nurse is different from the traditional nurse–client relationship. A more intimate relationship develops because of the home environment. The psychiatric home care nurse who is mature and understands the boundaries in a therapeutic relationship will best be able to maximize the benefits of the therapeutic relationship and promote positive change. A poor understanding of therapeutic use of self may result in chaotic outcomes and a destruction of therapeutic rapport.

Nursing care in the home usually centers around issues of safety and compliance. Increasing structure, using individualized behavioral plans, medication monitoring and teaching, role modeling, facilitating client connections to community resources, and working within the family system to promote healthy change are all important components of psychiatric home care nursing. The nurse must be highly skilled, enjoy working independently, and be flexible. The nurse needs to be creative, warm, and compassionate, but be able to set limits effectively.

The home care nurse is professionally isolated and needs to schedule time with other psychiatric nurses or a mentor for consultation and support. It is vital that the nurse meet with other psychiatric home care nurses or a mentor on a regular basis for consultation. Consultation offers constructive feedback and support while enhancing and refining nursing skills.

Psychiatric home care nursing yields quality results in a cost-efficient manner when done well. To promote this mode of care, outcome studies need to be encouraged to definitively determine success rates, patient satisfaction, and cost-effectiveness. Psychiatric home care is an important option in the management of the mentally ill. It enhances current treatment modalities and widens therapeutic options.

BIBLIOGRAPHY

Brenner-Carson, V. (1994). *Psychiatric home care manual.* Baltimore: Bay Area Health Care.

Burns, T., Raftery, J., Beadsmoore, A., McGuigan, S., & Dickson, M. (1993). A controlled trial of home-based acute psychiatric services: 2. Treatment patterns and costs. *British Journal of Psychiatry, 163,* 55–61.

Duffy, J. M., & Parlocha, P. (1993). Psychiatric home care. *Home Healthcare Nurse, 11,* 22–28.

Harris, M. D. (1993). Psychiatric evaluation and therapy. *Home Healthcare Nurse, 11,* 66–67.

Hellwig, K. (1993). Psychiatric home care nursing: Managing patients in the community setting. *Journal of Psychosocial Nursing and Mental Health Services, 31,* 21–24, 34–35.

Kozlak, J., & Thobaben, M. (1992). Treating the elderly mentally ill at home. *Perspectives in Psychiatric Care, 28,* 31–35.

Kozlak, J., & Thobaben, M. (1994). Psychiatric home health nursing of the aged: A selected literature review. *Geriatric Nursing: American Journal of Care for the Aging, 15,* 148–150.

Pellietier, R. (1988). Psychiatric home care. *Journal of Psychosocial Nursing and Mental Health Services, 26,* 22–27.

Richie, F., & Lusky, K. (1987). Psychiatric home health nursing: A new role in community mental health. *Community Mental Health Journal, 23,* 229–235.

Thobaben, M. (1989). Developing a psychiatric nursing home health service. *Caring, 8,* 10–14.

CHAPTER 16

Family Caregivers of the Disabled in Australia

Cynthia L. Schultz

In Australia, "a series of Acts and Reviews since the 1985 Home and Community Care Act have resulted in support for a move from large-scale residential care to provision of a range of support services to people in their own homes, or in smaller home-like centers" (Australian Bureau of Statistics [ABS], 1995a, p. 3). Home care involves dependent persons living alone or with family. In keeping with the ABS publication *Focus on Families: Caring in Families,* from which information of relevance to the provision of home care services has been drawn, this chapter devotes particular attention to the informal, unpaid family caregiver of persons with disability. The definition of *disability,* on which the ABS figures were based, was "the presence of one or more of a selected group of limitations, restrictions or impairments which had lasted, or were likely to last, for a period of six months or more." A *handicap* was identified "as a limitation in performing certain tasks associated with daily living" (p. 41).

The *Focus on Families: Caring in Families* publication described how community-based care of people with disability depends heavily on families. It was reported that almost three quarters (73%) of people with a handicap lived in families. It confirmed that women are the primary caregivers, but outlined the considerable contribution of men in this role. It was reported that "fifty-four per cent of all carers who lived in the same household as the person receiving care were men"; "sixty-six per cent of male carers cared for a partner, compared with 53 per cent of female carers"; and "forty-two per cent of all principal carers were providing care to their partner" (p. 2). In the *Family Life* publication of the same ABS *Focus on Families* series (1995b), persons aged 60 years and older who were living in a family were asked, "whether they could care for themselves if left alone," and "who would help care." More than a quarter said that "no one would help or they did not know who would help if all members of the household had to go away for a few days" (p. 39). Moreover, only 8% of older people stated that they would use formal services (p. 38).

CARER POPULATION

In 1993, 18% of Australians had a disability and 8% of the total Australian population of more than 18 million were carers who lived in the same household as the person for whom they cared.

There were more than half a million principal carers of people with profound and severe handicaps. Of these, 229,000 were providing care to a spouse, 151,000 to a parent, 89,000 to a child 5 years of age and older, and almost 72,000 to other family members (e.g., siblings, grand-parents, aunts, or uncles), or to nonfamily members (ABS, 1995a, p. 25). These figures do not consider those parents of children under 5 years of age with profound disability, nor those parents raising children with less severe disability. Of interest, given the large migrant population in Australia, is the finding that people had a similar chance of having their needs for assistance fully met, regardless of whether born in a non-English or English-speaking country.

Principal carers of disabled children or partners, 157,000 of whom were aged 60 years and older, "were more likely to report stress-related illness, worry, depression, anger or lack of energy than those caring for other people" (ABS, 1995a, p. 2). Moreover, "over half of all principal carers did not receive any help with the caring role from [other] family, friends or formal organization" (p. 39). Reasons given for not receiving outside help included lack of knowledge about available services or unavailability of same in the area, costliness, or "that the person need-ing help did not consider their need important enough" (p. 7). Twenty-eight percent of carers were providing care for someone in another household, and 20% of those caring for a child had been doing so for 20 years or longer (p. 28).

These figures, coupled with the fact that in the last 20 years the number of people aged 65 and older has doubled to 2.1 million, leave little doubt about the significant role played by informal carers in Australian households and the load often carried by families. Furthermore, a recent survey of 26,000 households in the State of Victoria revealed that carers differed from "noncarers" in reporting more health problems and higher use of medication; more feelings of overload, anxiety, and depression; less life satisfaction; and less support from other family members and friends (Schofield, Herrman, Bloch, & Singh, 1995).

HOME AND COMMUNITY CARE

With a federal government, seven state governments, and two capital territories, as well as local government authorities in each state and territory, the coordination of services and support programs in Australia—a country geographically the size of Europe—represents a major challenge. Fragmentation of efforts is inevitable, given the diversity and plethora of organizations and charities providing services and the variety of funding sources: private, church, business, and government. The Home and Community Care (HACC) Program, jointly funded and administered by commonwealth and state/territory initiatives, has gone some way to alleviating these problems.

The HACC Program was introduced by the commonwealth government in 1985 to provide generalized care and support services for the affected individual and the primary caregiver of targeted groups. Until then, community care in Australia was provided through four separate legislated programs. However, as pointed out in a Parliamentary Report on the HACC Program by the House of Representatives Standing Committee on Community Affairs (HRSCCA) (1994), it became apparent during the 1970s and early 1980s that the care provided under the Home Nursing Subsidy Act, 1957; the States Grants (Home Care) Act, 1969; the States Grant (Paramedical Services) Act, 1969; and the Delivered Meals Subsidy Act, 1970 "was not meeting the needs of frail elderly people and younger people with disabilities and the carers of these groups" (p. 7). Thus, the HACC Program was introduced to counteract the fragmented, limited, and loosely targeted previous services. The report further states that

> The Act brought the range of community care services for the aged together under a single umbrella for the first time, introduced a more specific focus to community care and expanded the target group of these services to include younger people with disabilities. It also recognized and provided support for the first time to those who care for frail elderly people and younger people with disabilities. (p. 9)

More recently, a special dementia focus has been introduced to provide information, community services, respite care, and research. Evidence given to the Committee on Community Affairs indicated the positive outcomes of the HACC Program. A range of services is provided, and family carers have been explicitly recognized as a target group. An income- and assets-tested carer pension is available, there is a pharmaceutical benefits scheme, and a domiciliary nursing care benefit is provided under certain conditions. The intention is to provide services that facilitate the prospect of members of target groups continuing to live in the community. These services include the provision of guardianship and advocacy, whereby caregivers are advised on ethical issues as well as decision making for adults no longer in a position to do so themselves (Minichiello, Alexander, & Jones, 1992).

The relatively recently formed National and State Carers' Associations are working toward dissemination of information to carers in a cohesive fashion, with Carer Support Kits being widely circulated. Training and advocacy programs have also been supported. Faced with an aging population and an increasing proportion of older people in the population, it is anticipated that the disability rate will actually increase. Thus, there is scope for the development of innovative support programs for family carers as well as the maintenance of well-established practices of proven value.

In summary, since the introduction of the HACC Program, the range of community services has expanded, funding levels have increased, and coordination and integration of services have improved. The Commonwealth Department of Human Services and Health estimated, in its submission to the parliamentary enquiry (see p. 10 of the report), that around 215,000 people use HACC services in a month. However, the committee concluded that "there is considerable scope for improvement in the structure and delivery of community care in Australia" (HRSCCA, 1994, p. 11). On support of carers, it was clearly stated that community care policies must facilitate its continuance and "must be cognizant of any projected changes in the availability of carers" (p. 29). Improved linkages between programs through consultation among the various levels of government, including local government, was also advocated, with the latter to be given "a formal role in needs based and strategic planning" (p. 198). Quality assurance was seen to be of prime importance in program development and service delivery.

CARER CONCERNS

On the basis of figures presented, it is estimated that as many as 1 in 30 adults in Australia are involved in providing special care toward close relatives, whether that person is a frail elderly parent, a child with severe physical or intellectual impairment, or a seriously disabled spouse. Frequently, people in these situations do not think of themselves as "carers" or "caregivers." Many see the loving care they provide for dependent family members as their privilege and responsibility. Unfortunately, this love does not automatically remove the inevitable physical and emotional toll that occurs. Perhaps this situation is best described as an unequally distributed labor of love. As much as the care recipient and caregiver may long for it to be otherwise, circumstances often preclude an equalized level of reciprocity and mutuality. Many carers speak of the "burden" of caregiving resulting from the demands and pressures—physical, emotional, spiritual, financial, social, and psychological—that impact on their health, family, and careers. Yet others express satisfaction that they are able to provide care for a person to whom they owe so much.

Drawing on the work of but a few Australian authors in the area provides some theoretical background and perspective to these circumstances. (For a broader coverage see Schultz [1994].) Braithwaite (1990) has identified five crises of decline for carers of dependent elderly persons. Awareness of degeneration in a loved one is painful to observe. It arouses strong emotions, leaving one feeling helpless; vulnerable; and, often, angry. The second crisis, that of unpredictability, arises out of the first. Finding oneself in a caregiving role can in itself be sudden and entirely unexpected; in other cases, it can be reasonably anticipated. In either situation, however, the rate of decline and the course of the disease are unknown. A day-to-day existence prevails, with the future often unpredictable. Time constraints are a third crisis faced by caregivers, one frequently exacerbated by the carer's life stage, which might entail a career, the raising of a young family, or personal frailty and decline in health. Finding time for oneself is perhaps one of the most serious problems facing caregivers.

The social and emotional relationship between adult caregiver and adult care recipient as a further crisis is well recognized in our society. The Australian *Mother and Son* television series clearly portrays the threat posed by the prospect of role reversal, and the loss of self, power, and control. Then there are those who did not enjoy a harmonious relationship before the one person became dependent on the other. Consider the anger and resentment of those who have little choice but to become the primary caregivers of persons whom they actively dislike. Lack of choice is the fifth crisis described by Braithwaite (1990). Given the strength of family ties, there often is little choice but to step in and provide care. This may involve putting aside other plans, a career, and favorite activities, and taking on new and irksome tasks. "Feeling trapped" is a common expression used by caregivers. The overriding factor for many is a steady losing of touch with self; absorption with the task at hand takes over and dominates their lives.

The inability to provide extensive care for a loved one because of one's own frailty can be a traumatic blow to self-esteem. Alternatively, it cannot be assumed that there will always be a willingness to provide extensive care. The "granny dumping," which Thea Astley (1994) described so poignantly in her recent novel *Coda,* points to an entirely different type of response. For those who are willing to provide an extraordinary level of care, there sometimes comes a breaking point, when the pressures and tension become so great that to their horror and dismay, they find themselves physically and verbally abusing the one for whom they are caring. The aftermath of guilt, regret, and depression is often intense.

Many similar crises and concerns are faced by those caring for disabled younger persons. Pressures in common may include all those mentioned and more, to which, in the case of the latter, might be added the unsettling undercurrent of hope or expectancy of recovery, the recurrent grief, and the lifelong care, which frequently places these parents in demanding circumstances far beyond those experienced in the average family situation. Recent research has shown that these parents experience profound and ongoing grief arising out of the fact that their child is suffering from an impairment, illness, or disorder that has long-term consequences for the child and for themselves (Bruce & Schultz, 1992; Bruce, Schultz, Smyrnios, & Schultz, 1993; Bruce, Schultz, Smyrnios, & Schultz, 1994; Bruce, Schultz, & Smyrnios, 1996). If the child was born with a chromosomal abnormality, or, if after an accident or illness, the child is now greatly handicapped, there was initial shock and profound disappointment. Subsequently, at important developmental stages in the child's life, the disappointment and sorrow are renewed when parents are confronted by reminders that their child will not attain the idealized image they may have earlier hoped for him or her. As Featherstone (1980) put it, "What fate should we mourn? There are a thousand scenarios" (p. 233).

The focus for the remainder of this chapter is on one particular innovative approach that seeks, by means of psychoeducational support, to prevent the escalation of personal hardship and suffering often experienced by those whose role is that of primary caregiver. The support is generic in nature, that is, it caters to caregivers irrespective of age, relationship to, or disability of the care recipient. Regarding living arrangements, the small group support programs are not intended necessarily to extend the length of time for which home care continues, but to support those involved in the difficult process of decision making before institutionalization and in the emotional upheaval that often continues after institutionalization. However, many participants in the program have been empowered to continue caregiving at home, having acquired a sense of control over their circumstances and being better equipped to handle crises.

Before describing the nature of the group programs and the system within which they operate, attention is drawn to some of the sources of pressure and emotions that have surfaced in these caregiver groups and have been reported more fully in *The Key to Caring* (Schultz & Schultz, 1990). The pressures may be of a personal nature, with feelings of inadequacy to meet the demands, self-doubt, resentment about disruptions to one's social life, privacy, time, or career; they may be due to practical and financial constraints, with apprehension about the future and how to make ends meet, how to provide adequate living arrangements for all concerned, and frustration resulting from lack of, or difficulty in accessing, community resources. Role reversal can cause considerable emotional distress—for example, the daughter having to be a mother to her own mother, or the spouse who no longer can share an equally distributed and reciprocal exchange of care as in the past, but must become self-reliant in all matters. Taking on a multiplicity of roles can also become overwhelming, as the literature on "women in the middle" has so aptly described (Watson & Mears, 1990). Difficult decision-making processes, disappointment over the deterioration (or little improvement) in the condition of the care recipient, and concerns about one's own physical limitations and health are but a few of the concerns of family carers.

CARING FOR THE CAREGIVER—SPECIFICALLY

Faced with a seemingly insurmountable load, it is encouraging to know that many caregivers have found renewed energy and strength, by being given the opportunity to focus on self through a *Model for Caregiving* (see Figure 16.1), which is now used in support groups for caregivers throughout Australia (Schultz & Schultz, 1990a, 1990b). The model demonstrates how, through awareness and a problem-solving approach, appropriate caring action can emerge. A triangle with three levels separated by broken lines has been chosen as a symbol of growth and to illustrate how the starting point is the personal, individual world of the caregiver—one's own self-awareness. Self-awareness includes what we think and feel about our daily experiences, how these fit into our plans and hopes for the future, and what changes are occurring in our lives. It is of pivotal importance to the preservation of self. As people get in touch with the forces that are at work in their lives, and the motivations that are important for them, a clearer picture often emerges of the issues that have been threatening to overwhelm them.

Support Groups

The prototype of psychoeducational support being promoted in Australia since 1989 is an example of primary health care in action. It has received funding from various sources including the commonwealth government, the Australian Research Council, the Uniting Church of Australia, and the Victorian Health Promotion Foundation. This approach is one of

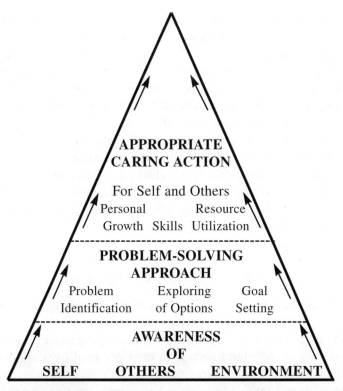

Figure 16.1   A model for caregiving. Copyright© Cynthia L. Schultz and Noel C. Schultz, 1990. Reprinted from Schultz, N. D., & Schultz, C. L. (1990). *The key to caring.* Melbourne, Australia: Longman Cheshire.

commitment to the equipping of people with special skills and insights, the strengthening of community involvement and action, and the creation of supportive environments. The system operates at three levels: (a) the provision of structured group programs for persons caring for dependent spouses, parents, and siblings, suffering from all manner of illnesses and infirmities, commonly experienced with advancing years, and for parents caring for children with disability; (b) the training through 3-day intensive leader training workshops of health care and other suitably qualified workers, who coordinate and lead the nine-session programs in their workplace or community; (c) ongoing in-service support to leaders, the constant monitoring of the program's effectiveness, and the publishing in professional journals of scientific evaluations of the outcomes.

The psychoeducational small-group structured courses, which are at the heart of this system of support for family caregivers, are known as "Caring for Family Caregivers," "Caring for Parent Caregivers," and more recently as "Care for Caring Parents." These courses are offered in the community through qualified professional leaders, with 300 having been trained to date and accredited to run support groups for carers. Group leader training manuals (Schultz & Schultz, 1990b; Schultz & Schultz, 1996) and textbooks for group participants (Schultz & Schultz, 1996; Schultz & Schultz, 1990) constitute the materials that have been produced after extensive outcome evaluation research to gauge the effectiveness of the interventions (Schultz & Schultz, 1990a; Schultz, Schultz, Bruce, Smyrnios, Carey, & Carey, 1993; Schultz, Schultz, & Smyrnios, 1994; Schultz, Smyrnios, Grbich, & Schultz, 1993; Schultz, Smyrnios, Schultz, & Grbich, 1993).

Course Objectives and Features

The courses share the same broad objectives, namely to:

1. Provide support for caregivers in developing strategies to reduce stresses in their families and in their personal lives arising out of their involvement as caregivers;
2. Provide insight and training to help caregivers improve their communication skills with other family members, the dependent person, health care professionals, and other service providers;
3. Assist caregivers to utilize community resources and to develop further their own networks of support;
4. Develop a therapeutic group environment in which caregivers can express and deal in positive ways with feelings and attitudes which may be adding to the burden of caregiving.

The courses have several features in common. They (a) provide structured, nine-session psychoeducational support groups that run over a 4.5 month time-frame, with six sessions at weekly intervals followed by three at monthly intervals; (b) adopt an holistic approach in addressing the needs of the caregiver group participants; (c) are based on the *Model for Caregiving,* which provides direction for the group process as well as theoretical orientation; (d) are generic (i.e., not disability specific); (e) are led by the same (trained) leader/s throughout; (f) combine didactic input with a maximizing of group interaction; (g) have specified goals and objectives for each session, with set topics for the first seven sessions followed by optional topics according to the particular group's preferences for sessions eight and nine; and (h) seek to empower group participants through the strengthening of their personal coping resources, the expansion of their networks of social support, and their utilization of community resources. While the educational methodology, underlying model, and basic human needs remain constant, there are marked differences in course content, as the authors consider it essential that the particular circumstances of different carer populations be taken into account.

A Model for Caregiving

The philosophy underlying the courses incorporates established theories concerning human behavior under stress, family functioning, group processes, family and eco-systems, and personal growth. It emphasizes awareness of self, others, and the environment, a problem-solving approach to life, and the development of inner strength and skills, and a wider network of support. The starting point is the carers' awareness of their own world—their perception of their experiences, needs, feelings, goals, pressures, successes, relationships, future, and so on.

The *Model for Caregiving* is designed to encourage the individual to take appropriate caring action, in the first instance, for self. This concept sometimes comes as a shock—"Is it not selfish to put my own needs first?", then moves on to relief at the realization that the extent to which you care for yourself is the extent to which you are able to care for others. Thus, it is customary to receive comments about the positive personal benefits derived by caregivers from working through this model in a supportive group environment: about being more favorably disposed to and affirming of themselves, and being more prepared to take time for self. In addition, outcome evaluation research has demonstrated long-term improvement in psychological health and well-being for group participants (Schultz, Smyrnios, Schultz, & Grbich, 1993; Schultz, Schultz, Bruce et al., 1993).

In making awareness of self the starting point, the broad phenomenological approach is followed, which claims that changes in behavior or attitudes are likely to occur only after clear and factual perceptions are gained and when necessary changes are made to distorted perceptions. By highlighting the necessity for the carer to be aware of others and the environment, attention is directed to the context in which the caring takes place. The courses include an important behavioral-skills component in the teaching and practicing of basic microskills for effective interpersonal interaction—listening, problem solving, assertiveness, and conflict resolution. These skills are applied to real-life situations and challenges constantly experienced by carers in their interactions with families, service providers, teachers, and other professionals.

As the Model diagrammatically suggests, the identifying and addressing of problems may result in personal growth, skills development, and accessing of resources more effectively. With clear perceptions of strengths and resources available to them, carers participating in the courses identify specific problems that need to be addressed, options that need to be considered, and goals that might be set, as they continue to provide care for a person with disability. The courses encourage carers to maintain, and where necessary to create, networks of support—among friends, family, social, or professional contacts. The courses not only provide skill building in creating social support, but are designed to foster a social support group among its members, not only during the 4.5 months of the program but into the future as well.

The Model, the group setting, and skilled leadership combine to encourage extensive opportunity for carers to address issues within the total context of their lives. This approach presupposes that carers, even when overloaded and stressed, are not helpless or powerless, and that it is both unnecessary and counterproductive for someone else (e.g., "the expert") to solve their problems for them. The carer will continue to face challenges and all manner of demands on time, energy, emotional stamina, long after the intervention has ceased. The courses intentionally seek to avoid the creation of group participant dependency on the leader. Rather, the aim is to teach insights and patterns of behavior whereby carers will be encouraged to develop even further their problem-solving approach to life. It is important that carers recognize themselves as having the power to identify their own problems, consider the options available to them, make decisions, and take appropriate action. When carers are reinforced in the awareness that they are responsible for themselves, their self-esteem and cognitive coping strategies are strengthened, and their sense of control over their own life is affirmed. Thus, by creating opportunities for competencies to be displayed, the concept of empowerment as discussed by Rappaport (1981) and Dunst,

Trivette, and Deal (1988) comes into effect: To be empowered, a carer must attribute behavior change to his or her own actions.

CONCLUSION

Much emphasis is being placed these days on the provision of home care and respite care for caregivers. It is heartwarming to note these developments and the government funding being directed toward this purpose. These developments are particularly crucial, given the deinstitutionalization process that has been occurring in recent years. External support of this nature is not only commendable but essential. However, there is a real danger that a disproportiate emphasis will be put on information giving and external sources of support, and that the significance and power of inner resources will be overlooked. It could be argued that one without the other is self-defeating.

To quote Ashley-Miller's prophecy in 1990:

> The 1990s will see growing demands for comprehensive care and support of elderly, mentally ill, mentally handicapped, and physically disabled people either in their own homes or in residential accommodation in the community. . . . Only within the community are to be found the involuntary and voluntary carers and helpers needed to supplement scarce statutory services. (p. 487)

Thus, in Australia as elsewhere, the implications for clinicians, practitioners, researchers, and educators are clear. How best to encourage and empower caregivers in the preservation of self, whether they are informal and unpaid carers or employed professionals, represents an enormous challenge. A combination and pooling of resources is imperative for the survival of a humane society. The need is compelling.

REFERENCES

Ashley-Miller, M. (1990). Community care: Research studies are essential. *British Medical Journal, 300,* 487.
Astley, T. (1994). *Coda.* Australia: William Heinemann.

Australian Bureau of Statistics (1995a). *Caring in families: Support for persons who are older or have disabilities.* (Catalog No. 4423.00). Canberra: Australian Government Publishing Service.

Australian Bureau of Statistics (1995b). *Family life.* (Catalogue No. 4425.0). Australian Government Publishing Service.

Braithwaite, V. (1990). *Bound to care.* Sydney: Allen & Unwin.

Bruce, E. J., & Schultz, C. L. (1992). Complicated loss: Considerations in counselling the parents of a child with an intellectual disability. *The Australian Counselling Psychologist, 8,* 8–20.

Bruce, E. J., Schultz, C. L., & Smyrnios, K. X. (1996). A longitudinal study of the grief of mothers and fathers of children with intellectual disability. *British Journal of Medical Psychology, 69,* 33–45.

Bruce, E. J., Schultz, C. L., Smyrnios, K. X., & Schultz, N. C. (1993). Discrepancy and loss in parenting: A comparative study of mothers and fathers of children with and without intellectual disability. *Children Australia, 18,* 18–24.

Bruce, E. J., Schultz, C. L., Smyrnios, K. X., & Schultz, N. C. (1994). Grieving related to development: A preliminary comparison of three age cohorts of parents of children with intellectual disabilities. *British Journal of Medical Psychology, 67,* 37–52.

Dunst, C. J., Trivette, C. M., & Deal, A. G. (1988). *Enabling and empowering families: Principles and guidelines for practice.* Cambridge, MA: Brookline Books.

Featherstone, H. (1980). *"A difference in the family": Life with a disabled child.* New York: Basic Books.

House of Representatives Standing Committee on Community Affairs. (1994). *Home but not alone: Report on the Home and Community Care Program.* Canberra: Australian Government Publishing Service.

Minichiello, V., Alexander, L., & Jones, D. (1992). *Gerontology: A multidisciplinary approach.* Sydney: Prentice Hall.

Rappaport, J. (1981). In praise of paradox: A social policy of empowerment over prevention. *American Journal of Community Psychology, 9,* 1–25.

Schofield, H., Herrman, H., Bloch, S., & Singh, B. (1995). *Health and well-being of carers: A comparative study.* Manuscript submitted for publication, University of Melbourne, Victoria, Australia.

Schultz, C. L. (1994). Annotated bibliography on family caregiving in Australia. *Australian Journal of Marriage & Family, 1,* 106–120.

Schultz, C. L., & Schultz, N. C. (1990a). As people grow older: Caregiving, health, and psychological well-being. *Lincoln Papers in Gerontology* (No. 5), La Trobe University.

Schultz, C. L., & Schultz, N. C. (1990b). *Caring for Family Caregivers: Group*

Leader Manual. (Available from Highfields Caregiving, P.O. Box 55, Ivanhoe, Australia, 3079).

Schultz, C. L., & Schultz, N. C. (1996). *Care for caring parents.* Melbourne: Australian Council for Educational Research.

Schultz, C. L., Schultz, N. C., Bruce, E. J., Smyrnios, K. X., Carey, L., & Carey, C. (1993). Psychoeducational support for parents of children with intellectual disability: An outcome study. *International Journal of Disability, Development and Education, 40,* 205–216.

Schultz, C. L., Schultz, N. C., & Smyrnios, K. X. (1994). Caring for family caregivers of dependent ageing persons: Process and outcome evaluation. *Australian Journal on Ageing, 13,* 193–196.

Schultz, C. L., Smyrnios, K. X., Grbich, C. F., & Schultz, N. C. (1993). Caring for family caregivers in Australia: A model of psychoeducational support. *Ageing and Society, 13,* 1–25.

Schultz, C. L., Smyrnios, K. X., Schultz, N. C., & Grbich, C. F. (1993). Longitudinal outcomes of psychoeducational support for family caregivers of dependent elderly persons. *Australian Psychologist, 28,* 21–24.

Schultz, N. C., & Schultz, C. L. (1990). *The key to caring.* Melbourne: Longman Cheshire.

Schultz, N. C., & Schultz, C. L. (1996). *Care for caring parents: Leader's manual.* Melbourne: Australian Council for Educational Research.

Watson, E., & Mears, J. (1990). *Women in the middle: Caregivers with a double burden of care.* MacArthur Institute of Higher Education, Campbelltown, New South Wales, Australia.

CHAPTER 17

Home Care Nursing for the Terminally Ill: Hospice in the United States

Elizabeth Ford Pitorak

Hospice in the United States, with a 20-year history, is a relatively new concept compared with community or home health care. As one looks at the continuum of health care, hospice, or care of the terminally ill, is the final level of care.

Hospice compared with home health care is different in philosophy and goals. Home health care is skilled nursing, patient focused, and rehabilitative in nature, whereas hospice is not only patient but also family focused and involves the use of large interdisciplinary teams with expertise in management of symptoms and pain—physical, social, psychological, and spiritual. Although home health agencies have dying patients in their programs, hospice, a unique health care delivery system providing palliative care for the terminally ill, is the appropriate level of care for patients and their families with end-stage diseases.

HISTORY OF HOSPICE

Historically, hospice care goes back to medieval times when there were way stations run by religious orders who nurtured and cared for sick and weary travelers returning from the crusades. These travelers sought respite and comfort at the hospice. In Latin, *hospice* means both host and guest, connoting the process of caring interaction. The themes of respite and comfort are dominant today, but the main concept is palliative care of the dying.

Dame Cicely Saunders of London, England, is credited for developing the present-day hospice concept. Trained as a nurse, later as a social worker, and eventually educated as a physician, she opened St. Christopher's Hospice, a 62-bed, inpatient facility for terminally ill patients in 1967. Today, the emphasis has shifted from inpatient facilities to home care programs. More than 60 countries in the world now have hospice programs. There are more than 2,500 programs in the United States.

While Dr. Saunders was establishing hospice in England, Elisabeth Kubler-Ross, a psychiatrist in the United States, began her work with the terminally ill. The results of her research, interviewing dying patients, led to the publication of *On Death and Dying* (Kubler-Ross, 1969). This best-seller contained a description of the U.S. culture's denial of death and the isolation that surrounds the dying patient as well as an identification of five reactions commonly experienced by dying patients and grieving individuals. The outcome of this research was the impetus for nonprofessionals and professionals to begin addressing dying and the reactions to any loss in a more open manner.

Initially, hospice programs were totally staffed by volunteers as there was no reimbursement mechanism available for care of the terminally ill in their homes. The Medicare system reviewed its budget and the cost of care for the dying. The results showed that a large percentage of money spent by Medicare was during the last 2 to 3 months of life when patients had frequent hospitalizations. In 1983, as a result of this research, Congress extended Medicare coverage to include hospice care and caring for the dying at home, which has provided some financial stability for hospice programs. The Medicare Hospice Benefit, a federally funded managed care system, provides per diem coverage according to the level of care—home, respite, symptom control, and continuous care. This model has been extended to a state level for those states who choose to offer a Medicaid Hospice Benefit. In addition, today many private insurance companies recognize the cost-effectiveness of hospice-level care and offer hospice coverage.

Hospice provides the same level of care to terminally ill patients regardless of their ability to pay. This is a unique feature not found in other health care delivery systems (Carroll & Graner, 1994). In addition, service is available for any age group, pediatrics through geriatrics, and any disease entity with a terminal prognosis including diseases such as cancer; AIDS; end-stage cardiac, lung, and renal disease; amyotrophic lateral sclerosis; and end-stage dementia (Alzheimer's disease).

In the United States, various models of hospice programs have been developed to deliver care. The basic structure for hospice care is home care with backup inpatient beds for symptom management and respite. There are four basic models of hospice programs: a free-standing community-based program not affiliated with any hospital or home care agency, a home health agency-based model with hospice as part of their program, a hospital-based program affiliated with a specific hospital, and a nursing facility-based program that provides hospice-level care for terminal residents. The organizational structure of any program is not the important factor but rather the quality of the care delivered.

Regardless of the model chosen, hospice-level care can be delivered to patients wherever they call home—their own home, assisted living, group home, nursing home, jail, or the street. In some states, there is licensure for hospice; therefore, it is unlawful for agencies to indicate that hospice-level care is being provided unless they are licensed as a hospice.

HOSPICE-LEVEL CARE

To be eligible for hospice, a decision to stop aggressive-oriented care and a prognosis of 6 months or fewer must be made by a physician. How the decision to elect hospice-level care is made can vary greatly. Usually, the physician indicates to the patient and family that all treatment options have been exhausted, or it is apparent that death is imminent. The decision to use hospice should be mutually shared among the patient, family, and physician as they will become active participants on the hospice team.

Hospice uses a holistic approach in providing care for the patient and family. Healing takes on new dimensions that extend beyond curing a disease. Among these dimensions are engendering hope (Herth, 1995), reconciling and deepening relationships within a family, allowing a person to die when they choose, understanding the special communications of the dying (Kelly & Callanan, 1993), easing the pain of dying, attending to details, listening to the verbal and nonverbal communications of the dying, aiding the expression of the patient's uniqueness, helping the patient find meaning to life (Frankl, 1963), assisting to heal the spirit, empowering the patient and family to establish realistic goals, and accepting that there is no right or wrong way to die. "For each of us, whether, patient, family member or caregiver, healing is marked by making a little progress down the path toward wholeness" (Mount, 1993, p. 37). Dr. Balfour Mount, who has done and continues to do outstanding in-depth work in palliative care, is a world-renowned practitioner, teacher, and mentor for those whose area of expertise is hospice care. The reader is encouraged to read his article, "Whole Person Care: Beyond Psychosocial and Physical Needs" as he succinctly states what makes hospice unique (Mount, 1993).

Care of the terminally ill is a specialty in itself because of these many dimensions of care. The specialty of hospice nursing, described as in-depth high-touch low-tech nursing, is different from any other type of nursing and requires a highly skilled and knowledgeable practitioner. Dobratz (1990) has defined four categories that characterize a specialist in hospice nursing: (a) intensive "caring"—management of physical, psychological, social, and spiritual problems; (b) collaborative sharing—coordinated and collaborated efforts of hospice care services; (c) continuous knowing—acquisition of the counseling, managing, instructing, "caring," and communicating skills; and (d) continuous giving—the balance of the nurse's self-care needs with the complexities of death and dying.

Interdisciplinary teams are essential to hospice care and are composed of physicians, nurses, social workers, nursing assistants, spiritual care counselors, volunteers, bereavement coordinators, and music and art therapists. Other therapies, occupational, respiratory, physical, and enterostomal, are included as needed. Bereavement coordinators deliver care to the patients and families in their residence. The composition of a team for an individual patient and family may include the physician, nurse, social worker, and bereavement coordinator, or all members of the team depending on the needs of the family unit.

Hospice is one of the few areas in health care that truly uses the team approach. As the members of a team work together and function at a high level, the team becomes more transdisciplinary with a blending of the roles of the various disciplines. The goal of hospice is to provide quality to life when quantity of life is limited by teaching and empowering caregivers to care for their loved ones at home.

HOSPICE AND CARE OF THE TERMINALLY ILL

In hospice, the focus is comfort-oriented care and quality-of-life issues. The unit of care is patient and family/significant others who become active participants in developing the plan of care with the hospice team. In hospice, the development of the plan of care and the delivery of the service according to that plan is the responsibility of the hospice team. In many home health agencies, the physician is ultimately responsible for the services ordered and the plan of care is the way in which the orders are communicated.

Important members of the hospice team are volunteers who have been trained in hospice-level care. The Standards of a Hospice Program of Care published by the National Hospice Organization require volunteer involvement (National Hospice Organization, 1993). If a hospice program is Medicare certified, 5% of hands-on care must be delivered by volunteers.

Twenty-four-hour availability of an on-call nurse to make home visits for symptom management and at the time of death is a requirement. Because of the complexity of holistic hospice-level care, the standard for nurse-to-patient caseload is 10 to 12 patients, a caseload that is much lower than in usual home health care.

Hospice nurses are known for their expertise in pain and symptom management. Pain management is the area of expertise that separates the hospice nurse from the home health nurse. The hospice nurse cares for dying patients in pain and repeatedly uses high doses of opioids to reach the patient's comfort level (Gurfolino & Dumas, 1994). Symptom management may also differ in hospice. The principles used in symptom management are dependent on the life expectancy of the individual. If the patient has months to live, a symptom will be treated aggressively. For example, if the patient had months to live and developed pneumonia, intravenous antibiotics would be administered. If the same patient was actively dying with hours to days of life, the symptoms would be treated with oxygen to relieve any difficulty breathing and medication to control an elevated temperature.

Bereavement follow-up with family/significant others for 1 year after the death of a loved one is part of standard hospice care. Some managed care systems, such as home health agencies, do not usually include bereavement services in the plan of care. Bereavement services include contact from a bereavement coordinator or other members of the team, bereavement/grief support groups, educational programs, and referrals for treatment of complicated grief.

PAIN CONTROL

Dying in pain is a universal fear. To control pain effectively in the terminally ill patient necessitates using a holistic approach in treating all types of pain—physical, spiritual, psychological, and social. Initially, pain manifests itself as physical, but other types may surface later. Patients do not usually state that they are experiencing social isolation or state that they have spiritual pain, which is decreasing their pain threshold and increasing the physical pain. It is apparent that the nurse, who has expertise in treating the physical pain, cannot effectively control the total pain without working as a team with members of the other disciplines who have the expertise to address the other components of pain.

The pain of cancer may be the most difficult to control. In 1994, The Clinical Practice Guideline for the Management of Cancer Pain was published (Agency for Health Care Policy and Research, 1994). These guidelines, developed by a panel of experts in cancer pain control, should become the knowledge base for all nurses and physicians doing pain control with cancer patients and terminally ill patients.

There are three common types of cancer pain: nerve, bone, and visceral. A detailed assessment is imperative to ascertain the characteristics of the pain as each type of pain has its own characteristics and is managed differently. If the correct adjuvant medication is not prescribed, no amount of opioid or nonopioid analgesic will control the pain.

In 90+% of the cases, cancer pain can be controlled. Usually it is not a question of knowing the correct pharmacological intervention but having all parties work as a team in executing the plan of care. To this day, fear of addiction remains a major concern with physicians, nurses, patients, and families, resulting in underprescribing and refusing to take the prescribed dose of opioids. Opioid tolerance and physical dependence will occur with prolonged use of opioids and should not be confused with addiction (psychological dependence) manifested as substance abuse behavior. To identify the incidence of addiction, Porter and Jick (1980) studied almost 12,000 hospitalized medical inpatients who received at least one narcotic. Only four patients could be reasonably well documented as being addicted.

There are two parts to the pharmacological control of cancer pain. One is using opioid and nonopioid analgesics, and the other is using adjuvant medications. By definition, adjuvant medications are those that were originally developed for another reason. For example, tricyclic antidepressants are the adjuvant medications used for nerve pain.

In 1990, The World Health Organization (WHO) devised the analgesic ladder for the rational titration of therapy for cancer pain. This analgesic ladder provides a logical sequencing of opioids and adjuvant medications as the degree of pain increases. The major principles associated with pain control are that opioids should be administered orally and given around the clock. It is a common misconception that opioids administered parenterally are more effective. The route does not determine effectiveness but rather the correct dose for the selected route. Equianalgesic charts are available to determine the correct dose for each route of administration. To illustrate, three times as much morphine must be administered orally to be equivalent to a parenteral dose.

Morphine is a strong opioid that is effective in controlling pain. It is usually the opioid of choice because it is available in many forms—parenterally, rectally, sublingually, and orally in short-acting or long-acting pill or elixir forms.

In addition to the misconception about addiction, health care professionals are hesitant to use high doses of morphine because of the fear of respiratory depression. However, there is no limit to the maximum dose of morphine. Dosing is relative to the individual body size and tolerance. As the dose is increased, the patient gradually develops tolerance with sedation occurring before any respiratory depression. The ultimate goal is good pain control so the patient can have quality of life.

ACTIVE DYING PROCESS

As the patient goes into the active dying process, which usually takes hours to days, physiological changes occur within the body. The patient begins to sleep more and have increased difficulty swallowing until eventually total inability to take anything orally occurs. Gradually, a degree of dehydration with an associated euphoria occurs (Rousseau, 1993).

Families require the support of the hospice nurse in understanding the problem of dehydration. In our society, food plays an important role as a gesture of hospitality, a necessity to heal from aggressive therapies, and a must to survive. Now as the patient is actively dying, suddenly food is unimportant. Associated with this confusion is the myth that patients experience pain if they die dehydrated. Some patients experience thirst and a dry mouth, which can easily be controlled with meticulous mouth care, but no pain.

Administering intravenous fluids to an actively dying patient creates added discomfort rather than providing comfort. As the cardiovascular system is functioning less effectively, the patient demonstrates signs of heart failure with fluid third spacing and edema resulting. The noisy respirations become worse as more fluid accumulates. This symptom is disturbing for loved ones to hear as they sit vigil at the bedside. Suctioning is not an option as the fluid is not accessible to a suction catheter. For some patients, atropine will dry the secretions, making the respirations less audible.

Families need assistance in understanding that no physical pain accompanies dehydration, and intravenous fluids will only prolong the inevitable and frequently do so without providing quality time. Teaching family members how to provide basic comfort measures for a loved one helps decrease the focus on dehydration and gives a sense of control in an uncontrollable event, death—as well as a feeling that they did everything possible.

Near the end of the dying process, patients may be unresponsive and unable to indicate that they are experiencing pain. If a patient has been on opioids for pain before the loss of consciousness, it is assumed that pain still exists. Also, it is imperative to administer at least a third of the daily dose to prevent symptoms of physical withdrawal as the body will be physically dependent. Morphine can be administered sublingually, thus avoiding the necessity to give injections (Pitorak, 1987).

REFERENCES

Agency for Health Care Policy and Research. (1994). *Clinical practice guidelines for the management of cancer pain.* Rockville, MD: U.S. Department of Health and Human Services.

Beresford, L. (1993). *The hospice handbook.* Boston: Little, Brown & Company.

Carroll, J. T., & Graner, M. E. (1994). Hospice is managed care. *Journal of Home Health Practice, 6,* 49–54.

Dobratz, M. C. (1990). Hospice nursing: Present perspectives and future directives. *Cancer Nursing, 13,* 116–122.

Frankl, V. (1963). *Man's search for meaning.* Boston: Beacon Press.

Gurfolino, V., & Dumas, L. (1994). Hospice nursing: The concept of palliative care. *Nursing Clinics of North America, 29,* 533–546.

Herth, K. (1995). Hospice nursing: Engendering hope in the chronically and terminally ill: Nursing interventions. *American Journal of Hospice & Palliative Care, 12,* 31–39.

Kaiser, L. (1995, November). *Creating a new future—pushing the edges of the envelope.* The Eighth Symposium on Healthcare Design. San Diego.

Kelly, P., & Callanan, M. (1993). *Final gifts.* New York: Bantam Books.

Kubler-Ross, E. (1969). *On death and dying.* New York: Macmillan.

Mount, B. (1993). Whole person care: Beyond psychosocial and physical needs. *American Journal of Hospice and Palliative Care, 10,* 28–37.

National Hospice Organization. (1993). *Standards of a hospice program of care.* Arlington: Author.

Pitorak, E. F., & Kraus, J. C. (1987). Pain control with sublingual morphine. *American Journal of Hospice and Palliative Care, 4,* 39–41.

Porter, J., & Jick, H. (1980). Addiction rare in patients treated with narcotics. *New England Journal of Medicine, 302,* 123.

Rousseau, P. (1993). Dehydration and terminal illness in the elderly. *Clinical Geriatrics, 1,* 32–36.

CHAPTER 18

Home Care Nursing in the United Kingdom

June Clark

The United Kingdom has a long and proud tradition of nursing the sick in their own homes. From the time of the Elizabethan Poor Law of 1601, the parishes employed nurses to care for the pauper sick in their own homes because it was less expensive than admitting them to the parish workhouse (Baly, 1995). The modern district nursing service, however, usually traces its history to the 19th century sanitary reform movement in England, which established most of the legislation and institutions that are the basis of the U.K. health care system even today. It is to this period, and in particular to the work of Florence Nightingale, that the establishment of nursing as a profession is usually attributed.

Although the name of Florence Nightingale is usually associated with the development of hospital nursing and nursing education, she was even more strongly committed to the goals of public health and home care. In 1867 she wrote to her friend, Henry Bonham Carter:

> My view as you know is that the ultimate destination of all nursing is the nursing of the sick in their own homes . . . I look to the abolition of all hospitals and workhouse infirmaries. (Baly, 1991, p. 68)

and

> Never think that you have done anything effective in nursing in London
> until you nurse not only the sick poor in workhouses, but those at home.
> (Baly, 1991, p. 69)

She also recognized that home care nursing required knowledge, skill,
and experience even greater than that required for nursing in hospital:

> The district nurse must first nurse. She must be of a yet higher class
> and of a yet fuller training than a hospital nurse because she has no
> hospital appliances to hand. . . . The doctor has no-one but her to
> report to him. She is his staff of clinical clerks, dressers and nurses.
> (Nightingale, 1881)

The start of district nursing services in the United Kingdom is usually
attributed to William Rathbone, a wealthy ship owner and philanthropist
from Liverpool, who employed a nurse called Mrs. Robinson to care for
his dying wife and was so impressed by her work that after his wife's
death he continued to employ her to look after the "poor sick" in the
surrounding area. Rathbone sought advice from Nightingale about establishing a proper service with properly trained nurses. Nightingale suggested that the Liverpool Infirmary should train its own nurses for home
nursing as well as for hospital work, and the first district nursing service began in Liverpool in 1863.

The idea spread. In London, the Metropolitan Nursing Association
was established in 1874; a Rural District Nursing Association and a
number of County Nursing Associations soon followed. The most significant development came in 1887, when Queen Victoria gave the greater
part of the money that had been donated to mark her Jubilee for the
extension of the work of district nursing. The Queen Victoria Jubilee
Institute for Nurses, which later became the Queen's Institute of District
Nursing, established a national training program and acted as the agency
through which "Queen's Nurses" were employed by the County Associations. The district nurse became a familiar figure and important health
care resource to most communities. Although her services had to be
paid for, they tended to be at least partially subsidized by the local
authority, and the cost to the consumer was much less than the cost of
a visit to or by the general practitioner.

SPECIALIZATION IN COMMUNITY NURSING IN THE UNITED KINGDOM

Meanwhile, other forms of community nursing were also developing. In many countries a "public health nurse" is responsible for providing all kinds of nursing care to people outside the hospital, whereas the United Kingdom has a long tradition of specialization in community nursing.

From the middle of the 19th century onward, while district nursing was developing as a service to provide nursing care for the sick in their own homes, the health-visiting service was developing as a preventative health care service, focusing mainly on the care and support of families and young children. Health visitors also visited people in their own homes as well as providing services in child health clinics. In recent years, health visitors have begun to rediscover and redevelop their original public health role, and to focus their activities on the community as a whole and on vulnerable groups within the community rather than on individuals and individual families. Their particular skills are in teaching and advising, and they do not usually undertake the nursing care of sick people.

The establishment of the School Health Service at the beginning of this century led to the development of the specialist school nurse, although this role was often undertaken by health visitors. The traditional role of the school nurse has been in activities, such as health screening and immunization, and the nurse's traditional workplace is the school itself. School nurses also provide advice and support to individual schoolchildren, and this often entails visiting them at home.

In recent years, many specialist nurses who previously worked in only hospitals have begun to visit people in their own homes. Sometimes they are based at a hospital and provide an "outreach service" to people in their own homes; sometimes they are based in the community nursing services alongside district nurses. The transfer of care for people with mental illness and learning disability from hospitals to the community has been accompanied by the transfer of psychiatric and specialist learning disability nurses; more recently, community psychiatric nursing and community learning disability nursing have developed as specific specialties. In the same way, the recognition that children should spend as little time in the hospital as possible has led to the rapid expansion of specialist community pediatric nursing. Community pediatric nurses care for many seriously or terminally ill children who previously would have been nursed in the hospital as well as for children with multiple handicaps and chronic conditions. Nurses who are specialists in fields, such as the management of incontinence, stoma care, and terminal care, also visit patients at home and act as consultants to district nurses on the specialist aspects of the care of the district nurse's patients.

The fastest-growing group of nurses in the United Kingdom is practice nurses—the nurses who are directly employed by general practitioners to work in the GP's surgery. Some practice nurses follow up the patients they have seen in their clinics by visiting them at home.

EDUCATIONAL PREPARATION FOR HOME CARE

Since the time of Florence Nightingale, it has been recognized in the United Kingdom that community nursing requires specialist post–basic education, and training programs for both health visitors and district nurses have been available for more than 100 years. Since 1981, such training has been mandatory for practice as a district nurse. Although many recently qualified nurses who have undertaken the new Project 2000 program of basic nursing education, which includes primary health care, work as staff nurses within the district nursing team. The UKCC has recently reformulated the standards for postregistration preparation for community nursing so that all programs will be at the level of a university degree, and all the different specialties will share a common core.

INTRODUCTION OF THE
NATIONAL HEALTH SERVICE

The National Health Service Act of 1946, which established the U.K. National Health Service, required all local authorities to provide a home nursing service. The act established, from April 1, 1948, a health service that was available to all citizens, funded from general taxation, and free of charge at the point of use. The organization of the services, however, did not radically differ from the previous arrangements. The service was organized in three parts: the hospitals, which had previously been run by various authorities, were nationalized under the control of Hospital Management Committees, which reported to Regional Hospital Boards; the GPs (family doctors), who had refused to join the new system unless their independence and autonomy were guaranteed, retained their independence through a system of contracting for named patients (those who registered their names on their "lists") directly with the Health Ministry; and the elected local authorities remained responsible for the provision of public health and community-based services including maternal and child health services, school health services, community-based midwifery, and home nursing. From the policy viewpoint, the difference was that services that had previously been provided through local arrangements, often by voluntary organizations, were now made the responsibility of publicly accountable health authorities and were to be extended where necessary so that all services would be available on the basis of clinical need alone, to all citizens wherever they lived. From the consumer's viewpoint, the difference was that all health services were now free of charge and were available to everyone. Thus, the local authorities remained responsible for home nursing services, but every authority was now required to provide such a service, and the funding came not from local taxation but as part of a grant from central government funds.

This system remained until 1974, when the NHS (Reorganization) Act brought together hospital and community health services under new Health Authorities that were established at regional and local levels. The local authorities lost their responsibility for health care (apart from some residual environmental health responsibilities) but retained responsibility for the provision of social services—a split that was always a problem for the achievement of coordinated community-based care but that was later to become a major problem. As in 1946, the GPs fought to retain their "independence" and continued as independent contractors. Funding arrangements remained broadly the same, except that the central government grant for all "hospital and community health services" (i.e., all health services except the GP services) was made to the Regional Health Authorities (on the basis of the size of the population served) who divided it among their Area Health Authorities (replaced in 1982 by District Health Authorities), who in turn used the money to provide hospital and community health services, including district nursing.

Although there were major organizational changes in 1974 and further adjustments in 1982 and 1983, the financial system established in

1948 remained unaltered (apart from the introduction of relatively small charges for drugs and some other services) until the major health care reforms of 1990.

NHS AND COMMUNITY CARE ACT 1990

During the past decade, almost every country in Europe has changed its health care system. The imperative for change in every country has been the need to constrain the rising costs of health care, and in most countries the core change has been the introduction into health care of the concept of the market: a shift away from the "public service" model in which services are directly provided by public authorities, to a "market model" in which services are purchased (often, as in the United Kingdom, by public authorities and using public funds) from independent provider organizations, such as hospitals or other health care agencies. This change is based on the "new right" political and economic theory that the introduction of this kind of market model, which requires provider organizations to compete with one another for the purchaser's resources, will improve efficiency, improve quality, and reduce costs.

In the United Kingdom, this "purchaser/provider split" is the core of the health care reforms that have been introduced by the NHS and Community Care Act 1990. The main source of funding is still public funds raised through general taxation, and the funds are still allocated to geographically defined public authorities (the District Health Authorities) on the basis of the size of the population served, weighted to consider factors, such as the population's age structure and mortality and morbidity profile. The key difference is that these authorities previously used this money to run the hospitals and other health care facilities in their district, whereas they now use the money to buy services from hospitals and other health care agencies through contracts. The District Health Authority is required to assess the health needs of its population, to use this information to specify contracts, and to buy services from the provider who can meet the specification at the lowest price. They may buy the services from the hospitals and other agencies in their own district that they used to run (which have now been reformed as independent not-for-profit organizations known as NHS Trusts), from similar agencies in other districts, or from private-sector organizations.

The main providers of district nursing services are the Community NHS Trusts, and the services are still normally provided under a block contract by the local Community NHS Trust, which covers the same area as the District Health Authority. From the patients' viewpoint, therefore, there may be little change: The same people are providing the same district nursing services, free of charge to the patient, to the same population as they did before 1990. However, the negotiation of a contract by the purchaser at the lowest possible price, coupled with the Trust's need to win the contract in the face of competition from other providers, is already producing changes in the form of reductions of some services, the introduction of new services in response to contract specifications, and various changes (such as the replacement of expensive highly qualified district nurses by less well-qualified but less expensive assistants) designed to improve efficiency and reduce costs.

However, district nursing services in particular are susceptible to a variation of this system which is known as "GP fundholding." Under the 1990 act, provision was made for some of the funds available for the purchase of certain health services to be allocated directly to GPs. Since 1993, the specified services include community nursing services. The scheme is voluntary; GPs who apply to become "fundholders" must meet certain criteria, such as a minimum number of patients registered on their "list," but certain financial incentives are provided. Since 1990, the scheme has been progressively extended to increase the number of fundholders by reducing the minimum required list size and to increase the range of services that may be purchased; "total fundholding" schemes, in which fundholders may purchase the full range of health care are under development. GP fundholders are beginning to use their purchasing power to change services. They may use their funds to buy extra services, such as physiotherapy or chiropody services, for their patients; through their contracts with hospitals, they may negotiate preferential treatment (e.g., shorter waiting times) for their patients; if they do not like the services provided by the local community trust (e.g., if they dislike the way in which the district nurses are managed), they may buy community nursing services from another community trust in another district. From the viewpoint of the patients who are registered with a GP fundholder, some of these changes are beneficial; however, there are risks because the GP's purchasing decisions may not accord with the District Health Authority's assessment of the health needs of the larger population, and also the power to place contracts with agencies other than the local Trusts may destabilize local services.

COMMUNITY CARE AND
THE "STRATEGIC SHIFT"

In addition to these changes, which are the result of the "purchaser/ provider split," two further policy developments have had a profound effect on district nursing services since 1990.

The first is the "community care" part of the NHS and Community Care Act, which began to be implemented from 1993. The 1974 NHS (Reorganization) Act had clearly divided the responsibility for health care and social services between the two types of authority; the new health authorities were made responsible for all health services (except GP services) including community nursing services, whereas the local authorities retained responsibility for social services. In 1990, the policy document *Caring for People: Community Care in the Next Decade and Beyond* (Department of Health, 1990), which formed the basis of the community care part of the 1990 act recommended that the "lead responsibility" for all community-based care should rest with the local authority, who, using the same "purchaser/provider split," which was also applied to the NHS, would purchase community care from the various providers on the basis of an assessment of the person's individual needs. The assessment should, where appropriate, be undertaken in association with health workers (e.g., where a person being discharged from the hospital would require continuing support from community-based services or where the person had "complex needs" that included both health and social needs), but the local authority would have the responsibility of designing and purchasing an appropriate "package of care"; this process is known as "care management."

A fundamental principle of the NHS as it was established in 1948 was that health care should be made available to all people on the basis of clinical need and free of charge to the patient. However, for social services provided by the local authorities, the local authority has the power to levy a charge; the level of the charge is decided by the local authority and, therefore, varies from place to place, and a means test is usually applied so that those who can afford it pay more. The result is that within a "package of care," which contains elements of both health care (e.g., district nursing) and social care (e.g., personal care not requiring a qualified nurse), the health care is free of charge, but the patient has to pay for social care. Moreover, because many local authorities have, in recent years, faced severe cuts in their resources, the level of charges may be higher than the level that the person is willing to pay. This situation poses great ethical dilemmas for district nurses, and also practical problems because of the time required for the process of care management and the complexity of the divided budgetary responsibilities. The problems of the district nurse are exceeded only by those of the patients and their carers who do not perceive the sometimes subtle differences between the health and social aspects of their care, and may be unwilling or unable to pay for services that they expected would be free.

The second policy development that is profoundly affecting district nursing services is the major shift in care from hospital to community settings. This change began more than a decade ago with the realization that many patients (especially frail elderly people and people suffering from chronic mental illness or learning disability) who were in long-term care in hospitals could and should be cared for in community settings. This movement, which has accelerated since 1990, is the cumulative result of several factors: the philosophy of primary health care as the focus of the health care system (WHO, 1993) and the specific commitment of the U.K. government to develop a "primary care–led" service, and the economic pressures on hospitals as a result of the 1990 act to reduce the length of hospital stay and to discharge people from the hospitals at a stage when they still need considerable nursing care.

DISTRICT NURSING IN THE
1990s AND BEYOND

More than 50,000 nurses in the United Kingdom work in primary health care, most of them providing nursing care to people in their own homes. Many nurses regard this field of nursing as the most challenging and satisfying because of the great range of practice and the professional autonomy that the nurse enjoys. There are many exciting developments, such as the Prescription of Medicinal Products by Nurses Act 1992, which gives certain community nurses the authority to prescribe selected preparations and dressings from a nursing formulary. New, innovative roles, such as the nurse practitioner, are being pioneered, and research is developing rapidly.

REFERENCES

Baly, M. E. (1991). *As Miss Nightingale said . . .* London: Scutari Press.

Baly, M. E. (1995). *Nursing and social change* (3rd ed.). London: Routledge.

Department of Health. (1990). *Caring for people: Community care in the next decade and beyond.* London. HMSO.

Nightingale, F. (1881). *On trained nursing for the sick poor.* London: Allen & Unwin.

World Health Organization. (1993). *Health for all targets. The health policy for Europe.* Updated version September 1991. European Health for All Series No. 4., Copenhagen: Author.

PART III

Trends in Home Care Nursing Worldwide

CHAPTER 19

Technology in Home Care Clinical Practice

Marianne Chulay

The use of health care technology has dramatically increased over the past 30 years. The use of drugs, biological and medical devices, and procedures have been used to improve clinical decision making and symptom management, provide early detection and prevention of illness, and enhance the individual's ability to provide self-care. Until recently, the impact of this technology explosion was primarily on acute care hospitals. Changes in health care delivery, though, will soon shift the balance of technology from hospitals to the home.

TECHNOLOGY TRENDS AFFECTING HOME CARE SERVICES

Emphasis on Cost-Effective Approaches to Health Care Delivery

The demand for home care services has risen dramatically over the past decade, with predictions for even faster rates of growth in the future. Fundamental to this increased demand for home care services is the movement to find more cost-effective approaches to health care delivery. The paradigm of where health care is provided is shifting from an acute care, inpatient emphasis to examining new approaches to health care delivery outside the hospital setting. Patients are moving out of the hospital much earlier in their recovery phase, and traditional hospital services are being provided in outpatient or home settings.

The emphasis on more cost-effective approaches to treating and managing health care problems will lead to earlier discharges from the hospital. To support patients' recoveries, many of them will continue technological support. For example, continuous intravenous antibiotics for endocarditis can be provided at home.

Expansion of Noninvasive Technology

Another factor in the shift of technology out of the hospital into the community is the increasing emphasis on noninvasive technologies to support physiological functions. Use of noninvasive technology will allow previously high-risk patient care situations to be safely managed in a home environment. For example, noninvasive cardiac assist devices and ventilators are available that eliminate the need for vascular access or pulmonary intubation to support failing organs. The continued development of these devices will increase the numbers of patient whose care can be managed at home until resolution of the underlying organ failure or transplantation can occur.

Computerization

Another factor is the integration of computers into all that we do. Home care will not be spared this revolution, with health care delivery and documentation being increasingly reliant on computers, facsimile machines, and connections to informational databases via modem. Bar coding pens can be used to scan bar codes rapidly for common nursing assessment, intervention, and evaluating phrases. The pen is later connected to a computer for down-loading of the information into a laptop or office computer.

Consumer Empowerment

Another factor affecting the use of technology in the home is consumers' desire for greater control over their health care management and the need for a higher quality of life than occurs during prolonged hospitalization. The provision of continuous intravenous drug therapy through indwelling central catheter systems with portable infusion pumps has allowed a variety of patients to be managed at home. Chemotherapy, total parenteral nutrition, vasopressor agents, antibiotics, antifungal agents, and analgesic drug delivery has allowed patients previously hospitalized solely for intravenous (IV) drug administration to be safely managed at home.

The development of relatively inexpensive technology for self-assessment of symptoms has greatly enhanced clients' ability to manage chronic diseases. Use of technology to monitor blood glucose levels (glucometers), bronchospasm (peak flow meters), oxygen saturation (pulse oximeters), and blood pressure allow self-management of diabetes, and chronic respiratory and cardiovascular conditions.

CHALLENGES FOR THE FUTURE

These changes in the health care arena will place new and additional demands on communities to provide support to home care clients with technology needs. Major challenges will confront home care providers in the future.

Developing and Maintaining Competence

The first challenge will be the development of competence with the new technology. Home care nurses, as well as the client, will need to develop competence with a broader array of technological devices than in the past. This will require practitioners to consider new approaches to education for the development of new skills and, possibly most important, for the maintenance of these new skills. This will be particularly problematic as the numbers of technological devices increase and nursing staff do not have frequent, repetitive opportunities to reinforce their own learning.

Suggestions to deal with competence issues follow:

• Look to professional associations that have educational resources already developed to assist practitioners. Some specialty content can be adapted to home care use, with little investment of time/energy.

- Have experts from the acute care hospital provide consultation on setting up the staff education programs. These individuals have been responsible for developing programs to maintain technology competence for acute care hospital staff.
- Set up a collaboration with an acute care facility where clinical experts with that technology would mentor some of the home health care agency staff. This is an effective strategy for maintaining ongoing competence with low-volume technologies.
- Set up skills fairs, where stations are set up to practice or test important competencies. Again, this might be done in conjunction with acute care agencies.
- Avoid large staff development demands by developing focused expertise among the clinicians in the agency. With this approach, core groups of staff develop expertise with one or two low-volume technologies. As clients require low-volume technological support, they can either be assigned to one of the nursing staff experts, or staff experts can provide consultation to the assigned nurse who does not have the expertise.

The challenge of ensuring safe, effective use of new technologies in the home care arena will require new approaches and ideas to deal with this situation. Now is the time to be creative and reinvent our business.

Supporting Technology-Dependent Clients

Another challenge facing home care in the future is supporting clients that are technology dependent for long periods. Finding cost-effective strategies for technology support, determining client/family needs related to short- and long-term technology use in the home, and developing supports for the client and caregiver will be crucial to successful use of technology in the home.

The number and types of community support services currently available will need to be expanded, with new innovative services developed. Suggestions in this area include 24-hour hot lines that provide continuous access to information about care-related problems, and telephone and computer linkages with groups or individuals who can offer knowledge and emotional support without requiring anyone to leave their home. Use of the Internet and other computer bulletin board networks could be instrumental in providing needed support to technology-dependent clients. Teleconferencing may also be an approach in the not too distant future.

New services and linkages need to be established to allow technology-dependent clients to lead as normal a life as possible—for example, finding resources in other communities that can support the technology-dependent client when they travel away from home.

Adaptation of Hospital Technology for Home Use

One of the greatest challenges the home care industry is facing is the need to adapt current hospital technology to the home environment. Much of the hospital technology is overly complex for home care needs. Many of these devices have several levels of alarm systems that may be necessary in a hospital environment but are redundant in the home.

It will be important to work with the manufacturers to develop less complex, sophisticated devices for home use. These devices need to be more user friendly for the non–health care person to operate. Without an engineering background, many people would be helplessly lost trying to decipher all the devices present on the models of hospital technology available today for home use.

One strategy to deal with this challenge of adapting technology for home use would be to develop partnerships with industry, so that home care expertise and knowledge of needed changes can be shared with the manufacturers. Various acute care nursing professional associations have used this approach and found these types of partnerships to be effective in meeting the needs of patients and families. Establishing opportunities to dialogue about the issues/challenges and sharing strategies and resources can accomplish a great deal, with little expenditure of money.

Another aspect of adapting hospital technology for home use is to rethink some of the routines for providing safe care. It is important to realize why certain safeguards may need to exist in the hospital but are uneeded in the home care situation (e.g., sterile technique for some procedures to prevent cross-contamination and built-in alarm systems to alert personnel in a noisy hospital environment).

It is important to consider how difficult it will be to teach patients/families to use the devices properly. Many technologies are complex and were never designed to be used by non-health care providers. How can education and support materials be revised so clients and caregivers can use these tools?

It will be important to keep these device complexities in mind when selecting equipment. The use of an enteral feeding pump may be relatively simple and easy for staff to learn and teach to clients. A programmable, portable IV infusion device may be much more complex for staff to learn and maintain competence with, not to mention the patient education challenges when you are dealing with an 80-year-old, frail elderly client.

Technology Assessment

Another challenge will be the appropriate use of technology in home care. Patients with sophisticated health care needs and technology support have limited lengths of stay in acute care hospitals, returning to home at a much earlier stage in their recovery process. Should their high-tech equipment accompany them home? The changing nature of the health care environment means that patients are leaving the hospitals and returning home at a much earlier phase in their recovery process, with many of them bringing their technology with them.

Nurses employed in home heath care areas will have increasing involvement in evaluating technology and its impact in the home environment. Rather than someone in the acute care hospital saying a patient needs *this* device, or could not possibly leave the hospital with *that* device, decisions need to be made within the context of the patient/ family needs and abilities in the home care environment. It will be important for home health nurses to be proactive in decision making surrounding technology use at home, acquiring skills in technology assessment. Facilitating the client's decision making surrounding the use of technology will be an important aspect of this process. The ethical dilemmas associated with technology use in hospitals will not be eliminated when these technologies are transported into the home environment.

Factors that need to be considered in evaluating the appropriate use of technology at home include: determining the needs of clients, their ability to deal with the technology, the level of technological support required, and ways the home environment impacts the patient's ability to support the use of the technology as well as the capability of the technology to perform in the home care situation. For example, changes in the methods available for providing IV therapy at home have exploded in the past decade, with many more new devices likely in the near future. Are these technologies appropriate for the home care environment, and if so, what factors need to be considered to best support our clients?

An assessment framework for evaluating technology and its appropriateness can be helpful in the objective and systematic review process. A framework developed for technology assessment in critical care could be easily adapted to home care use situations (The Technology Assessment Task Force of the Society of Critical Care Medicine, 1993). This framework divides the process of evaluating technology into several major categories.

- Safety and accuracy
- Patient outcome assessment
- Cost-benefit analysis
- Social impact

Factors for each level of evaluation are delineated and provide a comprehensive approach to decision making surrounding technology use (see Table 19.1).

In acute care hospitals today, technology assessment occurs primarily by committees that review products or medical devices for potential use in the organization. These groups function to make a priori decisions regarding technology purchase and use, using a cost-benefit framework. Mechanisms, such as this, need to be developed for home care situations as well as hospital-based use of technology. Suggested approaches for home health might include the following:

- Regionally based consortiums that could provide guidance for several home health care agencies.
- Informal work by experts in home care with dissemination to their agencies.
- Professional nursing organizations can provide a forum for these value analysis approaches. Many of these groups have developed research-based protocols for various types of technology. Clinical experts review available research and provide guidelines for clinician on the appropriate use of these devices in patient care.

TABLE 19.1   Components of Different Levels of Technology Assessment

Level I—Safety and Accuracy of Technology
  Indications for use
  Contraindications
  Potential complications from the device
  Bias and precision of the device

Level II—Effect the Technology Has on Patient Outcomes
  Survival
  Morbidity rates
  Patient satisfaction
  Quality of life
  Compliance with disease management
  Hospital readmissions
  Self-care capabilities

Level III—Costs and Benefits from the Technology
  Capital costs—equipment, accessories, and maintenance
  Frequency of use
  Improved outcomes/better patient management and savings over current
    system
  Education—initial and ongoing staff and client education, and their ability to
    maintain their expertise

Level IV—Societal Impact of the Technology
  Legal issues
  Ethical issues
  Political issues

Sources of Information for Technology Assessment
  Manufacturer's specifications
  Other users
  Clinical trials
  Meta analysis
  Consensus statements
  Case reports in the literature and Food and Drug Administration databases

Expanding Research-Based Practice

Finally, home care providers face the challenge of objectively evaluating technology use in the home. Research needs to focus on the impact that home care technology has on patient outcomes, quality of life, and the educational requirements of providers and caregivers. Additionally, cost-benefit data must be available to guide future decisions surrounding the appropriate use of technology in the home environment.

REFERENCE

Technology Assessment Task Force of the Society of Critical Care Medicine (1993). Model for technology assessment applied to pulse oximetry. *Critical Care Medicine, 21,* 615–624.

BIBLIOGRAPHY

Coalition for Critical Care Excellend. (1995). Standards of evidence for the safety and effectiveness of critical care monitoring devices and related interventions. *Critical Care Medicine, 23,* 1756–1763.

Hutton, J. (1986). Economic evaluation of medical technologies. *International Journal of Technology Assessment Health Care, 2,* 43–52.

Pillar, B., Jacox, A., & Redman, B. (1990). Technology, its assessment, and nursing. *Nursing Outlook, 36,* 16–19.

Richards, R. (1994). Interpreting decision-analysis models of cost-effectiveness. *Respiratory Care, 39,* 959–960.

Technology Assessment Task Force of the Society of Critical Care Medicine. (1993). Model for technology assessment applied to pulse oximetry. *Critical Care Medicine, 21,* 615–624.

CHAPTER 20

Quality Improvement in Home Care Nursing

Tina M. Marrelli

Home care can be generally defined as including all the providers of services and products to those individuals with health needs cared for in the home. In the United States, there are approximately 15,000 providers who deliver home care to some 7 million patients at a cost that was projected to exceed $23 billion in 1994 (National Association for Home Care, 1994). Home nursing care as well as other types of home care services continue to grow at a phenomenal rate. The United States Commerce Department has called home care one of the fastest-growing sectors in the health medical market (Weinstein, 1993).

There are shifts and changes occurring in the health care environment that have direct impact on home care nursing today. Managed health care, which increases demand for proven quality services at lower or more stable costs (Marrelli & Hilliard, 1996), is at the forefront. Managed care is a method to allocate the delivery of care while controlling quality and managing limited resources. The move to managed care is driven by three factors: cost, quality, and access. In fact, President Clinton's proposed American Health Security Act was an attempt to address these same three problems in the American health system. The effective demonstration of quality is the only way that home care providers will survive these turbulent and changing times.

Managed care is forcing health care providers, including home care organizations and nurses, to define the care they provide, cost account for that care, and demonstrate quality in the process as well as the outcomes of that care. These changes have contributed to the increased number of patients for whom home is their health care setting of the 1990s. Home care nurses must be prepared to practice in this new environment.

QUALITY: THE EMERGENT ISSUE
IN HEALTH CARE

Though some may view the term *quality* as the newest focus or only a buzzword of the times, quality is an important component of any health care service including home care nursing. Clinical competency, positive patient outcomes, and other objective parameters of quality are integral to the care and practice of home care nursing. Quality improvement processes cross language barriers, economic and social policy regulation (or the lack thereof), and myriad other geographic and cultural differences as well as similarities. This chapter seeks to provide information about some of the commonalities in home care nursing worldwide and focuses on one of these important aspects, quality improvement in home care nursing. An overview of home care and its growth leads to the need for, and the discussion of, quality. For purposes of this discussion, the use of the term *home care* will refer to home care nursing organizations.

ROOTS OF HOME CARE NURSING

There are strong historical roots for providing nursing care in the home. St. Francis De Sales developed an association of home visitors for the care of the sick and the poor. Later, in the 1600s, the Sisters of Charity were organized as visiting nurses by St. Vincent De Paul (Stanhope, 1992). Florence Nightingale and her far-reaching skills, work, and publications as reformer, nurse, and researcher was a pioneer in advancing nursing as a profession. Home care developed in the United States in the early 1880s. The Buffalo District Nursing Association begun by Elizabeth Marshall is credited with establishing the first Visiting Nurse Association (VNA) in 1885. By 1890, 21 VNAs existed in the United

States. In 1893, Lillian Wald and Mary Brewster founded the Henry Street Settlement in New York City. In 1909, the Metropolitan Life Insurance Company began to offer home care nursing to its policy members. Out of this payment system for home care services, the provision of services to persons other than the poor developed (Kalish & Kalish, 1986). The formal governmental structure for reimbursement for home care nursing services began with the advent of Medicare, which covers all Medicare beneficiaries, regardless of financial status.

MEDICARE: FUELING THE GROWTH

Medicare is the national medical insurance program for the elderly in the United States. Medicare was legislated through an act of Congress that was signed into law in the mid-1960s. Medicare is important because in many ways it has set the standards for the health care and home care industries. Medicare has developed conditions of participation for home health agencies that are designed to ensure the health and safety of patients (United States Government Accounting Office, 1994). Medicare generally pays for the care of patients (beneficiaries) who are older than age 65, the disabled, and those individuals with renal failure necessitating dialysis after being diagnosed with end-stage renal disease. This federally financed health care program has fueled much of the growth of home care and provided for a specific range of home care services to a segment of society that before this legislation may have been under or unserved. Medicare is the largest payer of home care services (National Association for Home Care, 1994). Not surprisingly, skilled nursing is the most commonly offered service in home care.

Medicare is a complex program that has evolved into a quagmire of regulations, manual updates, and congressional intervention. In the United States, it is known that Medicare and Medicaid generally limit the extent of tertiary care services (Keating, 1995). The discussion of the covered services is important because not only Medicare, but other payers or insurance companies generally pay for these same nursing skills and other services listed subsequently.

The basic "rules" for caring for patients who are Medicare beneficiaries are (a) the organization providing the services must be Medicare certified, (b) the patient is homebound, (c) the patient must have physician

orders for care, (d) the patient must be eligible per Medicare requirements, (e) the home care services must be reasonable and necessary to
treat the patient's illness or injury, and (f) the nursing care is skilled and
is provided on an intermittent or part-time basis.

"Skilled" nursing care encompasses 15 specific skills that home care
nurses provide and can be reimbursed for, when all the Medicare rules
and conditions are met. Briefly, the skills are (a) observation and assessment; (b) management and evaluation of the patient care plan; (c) teaching and training activities; (d) administration of medications; (e) tube
feedings; (f) nasopharyngeal and tracheostomy aspiration (suctioning);
(g) catheters; (h) wound care (which actually has three nursing skills:
observation and assessment of the wound, teaching and training related
to the wound and care, and the hands-on care of the wound site); (i) osto-
my care; (j) heat treatments (which is not generally used); (k) medical
gasses; (l) rehabilitative nursing; (m) venipuncture; (n) student nurse
visits; and (o) psychiatric evaluation and therapy services (Department of
Health and Human Services, 1995). These skilled home care nursing services are explained in lengthy detail and with examples in the *Medicare
Health Insurance Manual* in the Coverage of Services Section.

Besides skilled nursing, five other services may be covered if the
patient meets the eligibility and other requirements. They are physical
therapy, occupational therapy, speech-language pathology, medical
social services, and home health aide services. All of the individual disciplines have their own specialty-specific coverage and documentation
requirements.

HOME CARE NURSING DOCUMENTATION

In home care, the documentation must support covered nursing (or other)
care and demonstrate to any reviewer the care that was accomplished
and the plan and the movement toward predetermined patient-centered
outcomes. Clinical documentation is the written recording and demonstrating of the nursing process, based on the patient's individualized
plan of care, and movement toward patient-centered goals and positive
outcomes.

The interdisciplinary focus on quality efforts creates an incentive for
the entire home care team to collaborate and work together to achieve

the agreed-on outcomes (Marrelli, 1994). The clinical documentation demonstrates this collaboration through team meetings, case conferences, and other team activities and communication methods. From a payer or quality review perspective, the clinical record and the accuracy and content of the documentation reflect the care provided. For these reasons, the documentation needs to reflect compliance with home care nursing standards at all times.

FOUR SEGMENTS OF HOME HEALTH CARE

There are various segments or market niches in the overall home care industry. These include the durable or home medical equipment company that provides and delivers equipment, such as walkers or oxygen to the patient's home. Another segment is the infusion therapy or home IV care business. A third is the private-duty, home health aide, or personal care services organization; and the fourth is the home health agency (HHA) or skilled services program. Community health or public health agencies also may have skilled nursing programs and be an HHA. Home care nursing can be delivered through any of these organizations, but is predominantly provided through the home infusion, skilled services, or community health or public health organizations.

WHY THE GROWTH IN HOME CARE?

There are several reasons why home care continues to be the fastest-growing segment of the health care market. The following list provides a few of these reasons: (a) home care is generally a lower cost site than other health care environments (particularly costly inpatient hospital settings); (b) there is a continued paradigm shift from inpatient to outpatient and home care settings; (c) home care, under Medicare, has historically been cost-based reimbursement; (d) in the early 1980s, Medicare changed the reimbursement system for hospitals to a prospective payment system (called diagnoses-related groups) that encouraged hospitals to discharge patients faster to their home, while still requiring health care services; (e) advanced technology and its availability in the home; (f) population demographics including the increased number of elderly, the aging of the "baby boomers," and posttrauma patients needing rehabilitation or other care.

This rapid growth of the home health industry demands accountability for quality to both consumers (patients) and payers (health insurance companies or managed care organizations). The home nursing industry must be proactive in quantifying care, special skills, and demonstration of quality.

DEFINING QUALITY: THE ELUSIVE FACTOR IN HEALTH CARE

Quality is an important factor impacting home care nursing. Historically, quality improvement initiatives have been credited as the method that rebuilt and revitalized the Japanese manufacturing industry. The language of quality improvement is still evolving and terms include total quality environment, total quality management, performance improvement, continuous quality improvement, and quality improvement program. Quality improvement places the emphasis on excellence at the front end. This is another way of ensuring that quality is designed into the product (a satisfied consumer of services) and services (safe and effective nursing care).

There are various definitions of quality. A well accepted definition describes quality as a product or service that meets the consumers' needs, giving them what they want the first time free of defects (Demming, 1986). In this definition, it is apparent that quality demands that efforts are focused on doing the right thing for patients the first time, and that our systems and processes are designed to support these important efforts. There are four main principles in quality improvement: customer focus, identification of key processes to improve quality, use of quality tools and data, and involvement of all areas in problem solving endeavors (Bohnet et al., 1993).

Some of the hallmarks of quality improvement include customer satisfaction, a clear vision and mission, support across all levels of the organization for change and improvement, identification of key customers, the belief that the people doing the job know both problems and related solutions, and the ability to work effectively as a team.

HOME CARE NURSING QUALITY CONSIDERATIONS

There are a group of processes or actions that, though varied, have come to "look like" quality. Some of these processes include evaluations of patient care, customer or referral source satisfaction findings, effective data management, team member competency, positive patient outcomes (quantifiable goals of care), identifying the "best practices," benchmarking with peers who are perceived as the "best," effective communication and coordination, managers that "walk the walk" or demonstrate quality, and effective orientation and training for nurses new to home care as well as others unique to each environment. One demonstration of the commitment to quality for home care nursing is accreditation.

HOME CARE ACCREDITATION

Accreditation of health care organizations exists for several reasons. Home care organizations may seek to become accredited for the sole purpose of stimulating continuous quality improvement of patient care processes and services. As the managed health care model penetrates the health care system, accreditation may be used to differentiate between home care providers as well as to position an organization for the changing health care environment. Accreditation assists home care nursing organizations in the measurement of their performance in relation to nationally accepted standards. Accreditation is becoming an expectation or a standard in the United States as many insurance companies, which pay for the home care nursing services, want only to work with or contract with home care organizations that are accredited.

There are currently two leaders in home care accreditation in the United States: the Joint Commission on the Accreditation of Healthcare Organizations and the Community Health Accreditation Program. The actual process and work related to becoming accredited takes months of preparation, thought, and detailed follow-through. Accreditation standards promote the coordination and integration of quality health care delivery by all involved in the provision of care as well as administrative operations.

Purchasers (payers) and consumers (patients) generally agree that external evaluation processes, such as accreditation, should be more focused on actual performance and less on the readiness and capability to perform. Quality improvement initiatives are a proactive approach that seek to minimize the potential for future errors rather than focusing on the resolutions of problems after they have occurred (Marrelli, 1994).

DEFINING QUALITY BEHAVIORALLY

The following are some of the basic indicators of quality improvement.

1. Belief and adherence to a defined vision and mission
2. Provision of the right care the first time (having the right supplies, knowledge, assessment, and other skills)
3. Adherence to the home care nursing organization's defined policies, procedures, protocols, and standards of practice
4. Knowledge of and adherence to professional standards
5. Awareness of ethical issues and the process for their review or resolution
6. Accuracy in care and documentation to meet state, federal, payer, and accreditation standards
7. Collaborative communications with other team members for a multidisciplinary focus that is patient centered
8. Identification of new nurses to home care nursing practice and the mentoring of these new team members for success and effectiveness
9. Evaluation of care and process to improve the services or products continually
10. Teamwork regarding identified challenges that need the input of the members to identify the process and ultimately make recommendations for redesign and improvement
11. Benchmarking with leaders in the industry to improve a service or see how others better perform to improve performance
12. Ongoing review of the patient/customer home care experience
13. Data collection systems, management, and analysis skills
14. Knowledge and use of the principles and tools of quality improvement
15. Identification of linkage between care interventions and assessing the quality of the delivered care (outcomes)

16. Active participation in the quality improvement program
17. Identification and behavioral valuing of all customers interacting with the system
18. Others, based on the home care nursing organization's environment

COMMONALITIES THAT SUPPORT QUALITY IN HOME CARE NURSING

Though the structure, detail, and operations vary widely, there are a cadre of basic nursing-related tenets that are common to quality home care services, which transcend the diversity of geographics, cultures, and economic policies. These include:

1. Caring
2. Advocacy
3. Knowledge and knowing
4. Assessment skills
5. Interventions
6. Evaluation
7. Community-focused view
8. Family- and client-centered approach
9. Framed by mission
10. Complex and multifaceted care
11. Collaboration with others
12. Research awareness and activity
13. Identification of and adherence to professional standards
14. Awareness of limited resources
15. Holistic care
16. Others

WHERE TO FROM HERE: THE WORLD VIEW

Regardless of where home care nursing is practiced, a holistic view of compassionate care supporting self-care for patients will be needed.

The strength of clinical expertise, the structure of a chosen theory, and research-based decisions will contribute to a body of knowledge unique to home care nursing. Quality will be defined by our customers in this changing environment. The new information we glean and share from our practices, the identification and mentoring of new nurse colleagues, and the traditions of caring we bring to the challenges of balancing the cost-quality questions will all contribute to quality improvement in home care nursing.

SUMMARY

Although differences and similarities exist among home care nurses, there is value in reviewing what quality "looks like" to assist in sharing this information with other home care nurses worldwide. It is known through experience that when care is given compassionately, competently, and efficiently, it costs less. This satisfies everyone: the consumer or patient, the physician or referral source, the payer of the care, and the nurse who must deal with the reality of limited resources. Excellence in home care nursing demands continuous quality improvement endeavors, as this is a continuous investment in the improvement of care and services. Excellence or quality in home care nursing, regardless of geographic location, demonstrates nursing's accountability to ourselves and others.

Research and standardized research-based care are necessary for efficient and high-quality home care nursing. The continued expansion and growth of home care nursing will be the challenge for the nursing profession. In addition, the complexity of patient needs, legal and risk management issues, and emerging ethical issues as the cost-quality equations are addressed, will only heighten the need for demonstrable quality.

These endeavors will assist all facets of home care nursing including practice, education, research, and administration. There must be efforts toward integration of research with home care practice. Whatever changes continue in the turbulent field of home care nursing, there will be a need for clinicians who are skilled, competent, and compassionate who are guided by research-based standards of practice with a strong theoretical framework. These attributes and efforts collectively will contribute to quality in home care nursing.

REFERENCES

Bobnet, N., Ilcyn, J., Milanovich, P. S., Ream, M. A., & Wright, K. (1993). Continuous quality improvement. *Journal of Nursing Administration, 23*(2), 42–48.

Demming, W. E.: (1986). *Out of crisis.* Cambridge, MA: Massachusetts Institute of Technology Center for Advanced Engineering Studies.

Department of Health and Human Services. (1995). *Home Care Financing Administration: Home Health Agency manual* (No.11). Washington, DC: Author.

Kalish, B. J., & Kalish, P. (1986). *The advance of American nursing* (2nd ed.). Boston: Little, Brown & Company.

Keating, S. (1995). Health promotion and disease prevention in home care. *Geriatric Nursing, 16,* 184–186.

Marrelli, T. M. (1994). *The handbook of home health standards and documentation guidelines for reimbursement* (2nd ed.). St. Louis: Mosby.

Marrelli, T. M., & Hilliard, L. S. (1996). *Home care and clinical paths: Effective care planning across the continuum.* St. Louis: Mosby.

National Association for Home Care. (1994). *Basic statistics about home care 1994.* Washington, DC: Author.

Stanhope, M., & Lancaster, J. (1993). *Community health nursing.* St. Louis: Mosby.

United States Government Accounting Office. (1994). *Long-term care: Status of quality assurance and measurement in home and community-based services* (Publication No. GAO-PEMD 94-19).

Weinstein, S. (1993). A coordinated approach to home infusion care. *Home Healthcare Nurse, 11,* 15–20.

CHAPTER 21

Research in Home Care Nursing

Violet H. Barkauskas

From a practical health care systems perspective, it is believed that home care is a necessary and important health service within both developed and developing countries. Experiences in the United States, Lithuania, and several Asian countries have led the author to believe that, for most people, the home is the preferable site for health services and that institutions are acceptable and necessary as secondary and alternative sites for care. In many countries, the author has witnessed older clients who develop all manner of resources to avoid institution- alization—not that institutions are necessarily bad places for care; how- ever, regardless of quality, they are still perceived as being only second alternatives to homes, which, objectively, may sometimes appear less than optimal. The research literature supports this observation of prefer- ence for the home as a site for care (Barder, Slimmer, & LeSage, 1994; MacDonald, Remus, & Laing, 1994). Thus, because of the importance of the home as a site for care and because most of home care is nursing care or care provided by persons supervised or coordinated by nurses, nurses bear a unique responsibility to develop and use knowledge about this method of service provision.

RESEARCH THEMES

Several research themes have dominated the research literature in home care. These are the following:

1. Description of the needs of individuals for home-based, health-related services, the use of home care services, and the recipients of such services
2. Evaluation of the efficacy, safety, and cost of home care in comparison with hospital and nursing home care
3. Description of home health care providers
4. Caregiver issues

This chapter is organized around the first three themes. Space does not allow for a review of caregiver issues in addition to the other topics.

NEED FOR AND USE OF HOME CARE SERVICES

Research on home health care need and use has had three main foci.

1. Understanding of the factors affecting need for and use of home care services
2. Variability of resource consumption among clients receiving home care services
3. Comparison of clients using home care with clients using other types of care

Although home care is needed by individuals and families across the life cycle for primary, secondary, and tertiary prevention services, studies on the need for home care have focused on the needs for physical and supportive care related to illnesses. Despite this limitation in perspective, a recent large-scale study in the United States involving 42,000 households estimated that 3.2% of all noninstitutionalized persons need home care at any given point in time (Soldo, 1985). Moreover, individuals aged 65 years and older accounted for 58% of persons needing home care, with an estimated 12% needing home care at any given time (Soldo, 1985).

From research on the factors affecting need and use of home care services in the United States, we know that the following factors affect use and amount of use: age, sex, fact of recent hospitalization, type and severity of illness, type of care needs, living arrangements, availability of informal care providers, income level, source of payment for services, and geographic location of residence (Barkauskas, 1990). The old and the very old, the poor, and women are high users of home care. Those living alone and without informal care providers are also more likely to be using home health services. In addition to demographic factors, it is not surprising that those recently hospitalized with serious illnesses whose treatment requires frequent, complex care receive services more frequently than others. The final set of factors affecting use have to do with availability of payment for services and geographic area of residence. High geographic use is correlated with low percentage of married persons among the elderly, low percentage of women in the work force, low state tax capacity, high home health agency supply, high percentage of VNAs among all home health agencies, a large physician per population ratio, and a high percentage of Title XX funds (Social Security funds) for homemaker services for the aged.

Several researchers have studied interactions of demographic, illness, and care need factors for the purposes of developing estimates of resource needs and use for prospective payment systems and other planning needs (Saba & Zuckerman, 1992; Shaughnessy, Schlenker, & Hittle, 1995). Although insights into these various influences on home care are clearer, resource need and use continue to be a research priority.

Since home care is largely nursing care, several nurse-researchers have sought to explain and predict service use based on nursing variables. Nursing variables are difficult to measure apart from socioeconomic variables. However, a recent study by Helberg (1994) provides a model for the consideration of nursing measures and some evidence for their influence. Helberg created a nursing dependency measure composed of the following variables: nursing problems, nursing care requirements, functional status, and family coping factors. Nursing dependency, along with socioeconomic factors and medical conditions, accounted for 22% of the variance in number of nursing visits made and 20% of the variance in the length of home care nursing. Other nursing researchers have developed tools to classify patients according to level of care need (Churness, Kleffel, Onodera, & Jacobson, 1988; Peters, 1988).

The data presented so far in this chapter are from the United States. A recent multinational study sheds light on the possible differences in the use of home health care services among countries. Van der Zee and colleagues (1994) compared community health nursing in the Netherlands,

Belgium, and Germany on the variables of level of patients care dependency, the type and number of services provided, and the nurses job interpretation and job satisfaction. Investigators found that both the level of patient care dependency as well as the type of care provided differed among countries, with curative services being more common in Belgium and Germany, and prevention, educative, and supportive services being more common in The Netherlands.

EVALUATION OF EFFECTIVENESS

Because home care is a somewhat invisible component of the health care system (care is provided in patients' homes and observed by patients rather than in a health care institution where care is observed by other health care providers) but resource-intensive service, considerable research emphasis has been placed on the evaluation of its cost-effectiveness as a complementary service to other health care and in comparison with institutional care. Research focused on measuring the effectiveness of home health care services has been conducted with specific population groups to control for age, need, and treatment variables.

Preventive and health promotion home health services across countries are commonly directed toward pregnant women, new mothers, and infants. A significant amount of research on the effectiveness of these services is now published. Deal (1994) published a comprehensive literature review of the effectiveness of home-based, community health nursing interventions for the purposes of maternal and infant care. Her conclusions are similar to others cited earlier in review studies (Barkauskas, 1990; Combs-Orme, Reis, & Ward, 1985; Olds & Kitzman, 1990)—that home-based interventions by nurses are effective in promoting maternal-child health when interventions begin prenatally, target women in high socioeconomic risk groups, and provide intensive services to meet comprehensive client needs. The set of positive outcomes across studies is impressive. Deal's (1994) review and original articles cited in other review articles are for those writing proposals to develop or maintain services for high-risk maternal and infant groups.

In addition to services for socioeconomically high-risk families, several studies have been conducted on the safety of the home site for the prenatal management of preterm labor (Gill & Katz, 1986; Iams, Johnson,

O'Shaughnessy, & West, 1987), the postpartum care of mothers and babies discharged early after normal labors and deliveries (James et al., 1987), and the early discharge of premature infants who are developing well (Barrera, Cunningham, & Rosenbaum, 1986; Brooten et al., 1986). Results from such studies consistently demonstrate that the home is a safe site for such care, and that home care can be significantly less expensive than institutional care. Additionally, positive benefits have differentially been observed in the treatment groups receiving home care over control groups receiving more institutional care. These positive benefits have included improved long-term maternal-infant interaction, less pathology, improved health practices, and fewer social problems.

The safety and effectiveness of home care has also been demonstrated for children discharged with complex treatments, for severely disabled and chronically ill children, and as a parent substitute for working parents with mildly ill children needing to stay at home (Bosch & Cuyler, 1987; Burr, Guyer, Todres, Abrahams, & Chiodo, 1983). Additionally, the competence of families able to care for complex needs of sick children with home care support has been validated by studies conducted in the United States and Great Britain (Andrews, Nuttall, & Nielson, 1987; Athreya & McCormick, 1987; Emery, Waite, Carpenter, Limerick, & Blake, 1985).

THE ELDERLY

Most of the research on home care for the elderly has been focused on services for ill or functionally compromised elderly. However, the benefits of preventive home care services for elderly were investigated in Denmark by Hendriksen, Lund, and Stromgard (1984). These investigators studied the health services use and health of more than 500 randomly selected subjects aged 75 years or older living at home. Approximately half of the group received nurse home visits directed at enhancing self-care and scheduled at intervals of at least one visit every 3 months for a duration of 1.5 years. Significant reduction in numbers of hospital admissions, numbers of emergency medical calls, and deaths were noted in the treatment group. Calculation of estimated costs of interventions and savings provided strong evidence for the cost-effectiveness of preventive interventions for the elderly.

Numerous studies have been focused on the home health care needs and outcomes of home care services on sick and frail elderly, with emphasis on the costs and benefits of maintaining individuals in their homes and preventing long-term hospitalizations. The findings among these studies are inconsistent, probably because of unmeasured variations among subjects and interventions. Studies from the United States have demonstrated that home care for homebound elderly can be less expensive than institutional care for many elderly persons (Brickner et al., 1976); can be successful in reducing nursing home admissions (Gaumer et al., 1986); and can reduce numbers of hospital admissions and clinic visits (Zimmer, Groth-Juncker, & McCusker, 1985).

A British study (Currie et al., 1980) on the feasibility and efficacy of caring for acutely and subacutely ill elderly patients at home was conducted through a scheme of augmented home care as an alternative to hospitalization in an acute care facility. The findings from that study, involving 37 patients, indicated that functional recovery was more rapid at home than in the hospital, and that home care was feasible and acceptable to patients. Findings from another British study (Gibbens et al., 1982) of augmented home nursing as an alternative to hospital care for chronically ill elderly ($n = 24$) contained implications that (a) augmented home care may be more suitable and less expensive than hospital care if nighttime supervision is not needed or if such supervision can be provided informally, and (b) augmented home care is preferable to long-stay hospital care.

In an article that reviewed the research related to home care for the elderly published in North America and Europe, Chappell (1994) concluded that

> functional disability is a predictor of home care services irrespective of the developed nation in which it is offered. However it is now becoming clear that larger structural factors also impinge on the utilization of home care, such as the availability of alternative services, the availability of informal caregivers, and coordination or lack thereof in the system. The outcome studies have concluded by and large that home care is not necessarily less costly or better for the quality of life for its clients than is institutional care and have led to an explicit questioning of the objective of home care. There are not adequate studies assessing the long-range preventive potential of home care (pp. 119–120).

SELECTED PATIENT PROBLEMS

Several studies have been conducted on the safety and acceptability of home care as an alternative site for selected interventions. Through such studies the safety of high-technology interventions, such as home intravenous therapy (Niewig, Greidanus, & de Vries, 1987; Sheldon & Bender, 1994; Stiver, Trosky, Cote, & Oruck, 1982) and home oxygen and ventilator therapy (Make & Gilmartin, 1986; Medical Research Council Working Party, 1981) have been documented. The findings of other studies provide evidence for the efficacy of home care for persons with disabling pulmonary diseases, pressure sores, and diabetic patients.

Several British researchers (Hill, Hampton, & Mitchell, 1978, 1979) conducted a 4-year randomized trial comparing home versus hospital management of patients with suspected myocardial infarction. A total of 364 patients were assigned randomly to either home or hospital management of their acute myocardial infarction after intensive emergency care in the home. A 6-week follow-up of all study patients showed that mortality was similar between groups.

Studies on the effects of home care with patients after cerebral vascular accidents, and patients with terminal cancer (Gurfolino & Dumas, 1994), orthopedic problems, and hypertension have produced mixed results relating to improved outcomes and reduced costs over hospital care or no home care. However, in all studies, although home care directed to patients needing high technology or specialized services may not have demonstrated significant cost savings or improved outcomes, the home has proven to be a safe and acceptable, if not preferable, site for care.

NURSE PROVIDERS

Much of the research presented in this book has been about the education and additional preparation of home health care nurse providers. Although the author does not strongly encourage research on nurses, an exception related to home care, as nurses substantially affect decisions regarding recipients of home care and the services provided, is made. Additionally, the invisible and isolated nature of the work create unique need for the understanding of competency development and job satisfaction issues.

Various investigators have studied home health care nurse job stresses and their potential effects, assessments of competencies, confidence in working with ethnically diverse populations, and specific treatments and assessments (Bernal & Froman, 1987; Clarke, Goggin, Webber-Jones, Vacek, & Aderholdt, 1986; Schulze & Koerner, 1987; Stanek, 1987; Von Windeguth, Urbano, Hayes, & Martyn, 1988). Findings from such studies consistently demonstrate the need for initial, special orientation for nurses hired into home care and for continuing education for home care nurses. These studies serve as reminders that home care requires many of the same skills, but also special additional skills, to those required for care in institutions.

In an attempt to learn more about the decision making of home care nurses as related to maintaining or terminating services to clients, Feldman and colleagues (1993) studied factors related to selection of clients for longer duration of services and decisions of nurses about client discharge in a public home care agency in the United States. The findings from this study indicated that nurses make different decisions about the discharge of home care patients based on several situational variables, which seemed to have greater influence on decision making than agency policy. In discussing the findings from this study, the authors point out that it is difficult for an agency to evaluate the outcomes of its services if nurses do not consistently follow established agency policy and procedure.

SUMMARY

The foci of home care research reflect a collage of the multiple and diverse client groups served by professional nurses. The consistency of positive findings in several studies across client groups and problems is evidence of the probable existence of a unique treatment effect for home care intervention.

The research in home care contains documentation of the need for home care services and their effectiveness across diverse population groups including patients as well as their caregivers. Evidence exists that the ill elderly will continue to be the major client group for home care services. However, researchers have also documented the relevance and effectiveness of home-based preventive, acute care, and chronic care services for individuals across the life span.

Through use studies, investigators have sought to differentiate the users of home care services from nonusers or users of potentially more expensive sources of care, for example, nursing homes, and to determine factors associated with the amount of home care services received. Research has focused primarily on the elderly because of their high service use and because of the availability of use data from the Medicare program in the United States. Findings across use studies have been generally consistent, with the following factors demonstrating influence on the use of home care services: geographic residence, functional status, sex, economic situation, recent medical history, and living arrangements.

Once a patient is admitted to services, the amount of care received is affected by treatment needs, referral source, source of care, type of payment, and living arrangements. Nursing home patients have been shown to differ from home care patients in the dimensions of age and functional status, with nursing home patients generally being significantly older and more disabled.

Research on home care for disease prevention and health maintenance goals has demonstrated consistently that long-term home care provided to high-risk clients can be effective in decreasing risk and preventing untoward outcomes for significant percentages of individuals, whereas there is no evidence of effectiveness of low-intensity home care with low-risk populations. However, it can be argued that intervention with high-risk individuals is really a form of secondary prevention, or early treatment, rather than primary prevention.

The high cost of institutional care and emphasis on cost-containment have stimulated experimentation in early discharge from acute care facilities as well as avoidance of admission to them. The following conclusions can be derived from the review of studies on use of the home as an alternative site for individuals experiencing acute care needs, the terminally ill, and children with serious chronic illnesses:

1. A variety of treatments and care regimens can be provided safely at home by formal and informal caregivers and by the patients themselves.
2. In addition to being less expensive than hospital care, home care is usually more acceptable to patients and families.

3. Patients and families often have unmet needs for information, guidance, and assistance with coping strategies during their transition from acute care facilities to home and across the phases of care at home.

Findings across studies of the effectiveness of home-based health maintenance care to chronically ill elderly are inconsistent, probably because of sample differences and diverse measurement approaches represented across studies. Also, the predominant dependent variable of interest in these studies has been cost-containment through prevention of both acute care and long-term care hospitalization with some, but insufficient, attention to quality-of-life and other dependent variables. Two well-controlled studies have demonstrated contradictory findings about the cost-effectiveness of special home care services (Hughes et al., 1984, 1987; Zimmer et al., 1985).

FUTURE RESEARCH DIRECTIONS

Misener, Watkins, and Ossege (1994) used a modified Delphi survey to identify research questions and priorities in public health nursing based on the perceived needs of practicing public health nurses. The responses converged on three major research themes.

1. Client outcomes in the domain of maternal and child health and family planning
2. Maximization of effective client outcomes in home health services with emphasis on compliance, complications, and discharge planning
3. Recruitment, retention, job satisfaction, and image

Given that home care is a very general label for an intervention, and that content of home care services was not well measured in any of the studies cited, there is a clear need for a common taxonomy for both nursing diagnoses and interventions. A recent article by Moorhead, McCloskey, and Bulechek (1993) reviews the taxonomies for intervention measurement in community health nursing and proposes some approaches for the integration of taxonomies into research.

Although the attempt to understand the variables affecting the use of services has been substantive and provided insights into demographic variables influencing resource consumption, substantial unexplained variability in service use exists among patients with similar characteristics. Research into use issues in this field is still needed, especially with the current emphases on case management and critical pathways.

In conclusion, although the idea of collaborative research is not new (Henry et al., 1992), the author encourages the partnership of clinical staff and academic faculty in addressing the critical issues in the field.

REFERENCES

Andrews, M. M., Nuttall, P. R., & Nielson, D. W. (1987). Home apnea monitoring in the Intermountain West. *Journal of Pediatric Health Care, 1,* 255–260.

Athreya, B. H., & McCormick, M. C. (1987). Impact of chronic illness on families. *Rheumatic Disease Clinics of North America, 13,* 123–131.

Barder, L., Slimmer, L., & LeSage, J. (1994). Depression and issues of control among elderly people in health care settings. *Journal of Advanced Nursing, 29,* 597–604.

Barkauskas, V. H. (1990). Home health care. *Annual Review of Nursing Research, 8,* 103–132.

Barrera, M. E., Cunningham, C. E., & Rosenbaum, P. L. (1986). Low birth weight and home intervention strategies: Preterm infants. *Journal of Developmental and Behavioral Pediatrics, 7,* 361–366.

Bernal, H., & Froman, R. (1987). The confidence of community health nurses in caring for ethnically diverse populations. *Image: Journal of Nursing Scholarship, 19,* 201–203.

Bosch, J. D., & Cuyler, J. P. (1987). Home care of the pediatric tracheostomy: Our experience. *The Journal of Ortholaryngology, 16,* 120–122.

Brickner, P. W., Janeski, J. F., Rich, G., Duque, T., Starita, L., LaRocco, R., Flannery, T., & Werlin, S. (1976). Home maintenance for the home-bound aged. *The Gerontologist, 16,* 25–29.

Brooten, D., Kumar, S., Brown, L. P., Butts, P., Finkler, S. A., Blakewell-Sachs, S., Gibbons, A., & Delivoria-Papadopoulos, M. (1986). A randomized clinical trial of early hospital discharge and home follow-up of very-low-birthweight infants. *New England Journal of Medicine, 315,* 934–939.

Burr, B. H., Guyer, B., Todres, I. D., Abrahams, B., & Chiodo, T. (1983). Home care for children on respirators. *New England Journal of Medicine, 309,* 1319–1323.

Chappell, N. L. (1994). Home care research: What does it tell us? *The Gerontologist. 34,* 116–120.

Churness, V. H., Kleffel, D., Onodera, M. L., & Jacobson, J. (1988). Reliability and validity testing of a home health patient classification system. *Public Health Nursing, 3,* 135–139.

Clarke, J. H., Goggin, J. E., Webber-Jones, J. E., Vacek, P. M., & Aderholdt, S. (1986). Educating rural home health care nurses in respiratory assessment: An evaluation study. *Public Health Nursing, 3,* 101–110.

Combs-Orme, T., Reis, J., & Ward, L. D. (1985). Effectiveness of home visits by public health nurses in maternal and child health: An empirical review, *Public Health Reports, 100,* 490–499.

Currie, C. T., Burley, L. E., Doull, C., Ravetz, C., Smith, R. G., & Williamson, J. (1980). A scheme of augmented home care for acutely and subacutely ill elderly patients: Report on pilot study. *Age and Aging, 9,* 173–180.

Deal, L. W. (1994). The effectiveness of community health nursing interventions: A literature review. *Public Health Nursing, 11,* 315–323.

Emery, J. L., Waite, A. J., Carpenter, R. G., Limerick, S. R., & Blake, D. (1985). Apnea monitors compared with weighing scales for siblings after cot death. *Archives of Diseases of Children, 60,* 1055–1060.

Feldman, C., Olberding, L., Shortridge, L., Toole, K., & Zappin, P. (1993). Decision-making in case management of home healthcare clients. *Journal of Nursing Administration, 23,* 33–38.

Gaumer, G. L., Birnbaum, H., Pratter, F., Burke, R., Franklin, S., & Ellingson-Otto, K. (1986). Impact of the New York Long-Term Home Health Care Program. *Medical Care, 24,* 641–653.

Gibbens, F. J., Lee, M., Davison, P. R., O'Sullivan, P., Hutchinson, M., Murphy, D. R., & Ugwu, C. N. (1982). Augmented home nursing as an alternative to hospital care for chronic elderly invalids. *British Medical Journal, 284,* 330–333.

Gill, P. J., & Katz, M. (1986). Early detection of preterm labor: Ambulatory home monitoring of uterine activity. *Journal of Gynecologic and Neonatal Nursing, 15,* 439–442.

Gurfolino, V., & Dumas, L. (1994). Hospice nursing: The concept of palliative care. *Nursing Clinics of North America, 29,* 533–546.

Helberg, J. L. (1994). Use of home care nursing resources by the elderly. *Public Health Nursing, 11,* 104–112.

Hendriksen, C., Lund, E., & Stomgard, R. (1984). Consequences of assessment and intervention among elderly people: A three year randomized controlled trial. *British Medical Journal, 289,* 1522–1524.

Henry, V., Schmitz, K., Reif, L., & Rudie, P. (1992). Collaboration: Integrating practice and research in public health nursing. *Public Health Nursing, 9,* 218–222.

Hill, J. D., Hampton, J. R., & Mitchell, J. R. A. (1978). A randomized trial of home-versus-hospital management for patients with suspected myocardial infarction. *The Lancet, 1,* 837–841.

Hill, J. D., Hampton, J. R., & Mitchell, J. R. A. (1979). Home or hospital for myocardial infarction: Who cares? *American Heart Journal, 98,* 545–547.

Hughes, S. L., Cordray, D. S., & Spiker, V. A. (1984). Evaluation of a long-term home care program. *Medical Care, 22,* 460–475.

Hughes, S. L., Manheim, L. M., Edelman, P. L., & Conrad, K. J. (1987). Impact of long-term home care on hospital and nursing home use and cost. *Health Services Research, 22,* 19–47.

Iams, J. D., Johnson, F. F., O'Shaughnessy, R. W., & West, L. C. (1987). A prospective random trial of home uterine activity monitoring in pregnancies at increased risk of preterm labor. *American Journal of Obstetrics and Gynecology, 157,* 638–643.

James, M. L., Hudson, C. N., Gebski, V. J., Browne, L. H., Andrews, G. R., Crisp, S. E., Palmer, D., & Beresford, J. L. (1987). An evaluation of planned early postnatal transfer home with nursing support. *Medical Journal of Australia, 147,* 434–438.

Make, B. J., & Gilmartin, M. E. (1986). Rehabilitation and home care for ventilator-assisted individuals. *Clinics in Chest Medicine, 7,* 679–691.

MacDonald, M., Remus, G., & Laing, G. (1994). The link between housing and health in the elderly. *Journal of Gerontological Nursing, 20,* 5–10.

Medical Research Council Working Party. (1981). Long term domiciliary oxygen therapy with chronic hypoxic cor pulmonale complicating chronic bronchitis and emphysema. *The Lancet, 1,* 681–685.

Misener, T. R., Watkins, J. G., & Ossege, J. (1994). Public health nursing research priorities: A collaborative Delphi study. *Public Health Nursing, 11,* 66–74.

Moorhead, S. A., McCloskey, J. C., & Bulechek, G. M. (1993). Nursing interventions classification: A comparison with the Omaha System and the Home Healthcare Classification. *Journal of Nursing Administration, 23,* 23–29.

Niewig, R., Greidanus, J., & de Vries, E. G. E. (1987). A patient education program for a continuous infusion regimen on an outpatient basis. *Cancer Nursing, 10,* 177–182.

Olds, D. L., & Kitzman, H. (1990). Can home visitation improve the health of women and children at environmental risk? *Pediatrics, 86,* 108–116.

Peters, D. A. (1988). Development of a Community Health Intensity Rating Scale. *Nursing Research, 37,* 202–207.

Saba, V. K., & Zuckerman, A. F. (1992). A home health classification method. *Caring, 1,* 27–37.

Schulze, M. W., & Koerner, B. L. (1987). Attitudes of community health nurses toward maternal and child health nursing: Development of an instrument. *Journal of Professional Nursing, 3,* 347–353.

Shaughnessy, P. W., Schlenker, R. E., & Hittle, D. F. (1995). Case mix of home health patients under capitated and fee for service payment. *Health Services Research, 30,* 79–113.

Sheldon, P., & Bender, M. (1994). High-technology in home care: An overview of intravenous therapy. *Nursing Clinics of North America, 29,* 507–519.

Soldo, B. J. (1985). In-home services for the dependent elderly. *Research on Aging, 7,* 281–304.

Stanek, L. M. (1987). An analysis of professional nurse burnout in two selected nursing care settings, *Journal of Nursing Administration, 17,* 3, 29.

Stiver, H. G., Trosky, S. K., Cote, D. D., & Oruck, J. L. (1982). Self-administration of intravenous antibiotics: An efficient, cost-effective home care program. *Canadian Medical Association Journal, 127,* 207–211.

Van der Zee, J., Kramer, K., Derksen, A., Kerkstra, A., & Stevens. F. C. J. (1994). Community nursing in Belgium, Germany and the Netherlands. *Journal of Advanced Nursing, 20,* 791–801.

von Windeguth, B., Urbano, M. T., Hayes, J. S., & Martyn, K. K. (1988). Analysis of infant risk factors documented by public health nurses. *Public Health Nursing, 5,* 165–169.

Zimmer, J. G., Groth-Juncker, A., & McCusker, J. (1985). A randomized controlled study of a home health care team. *American Journal of Public Health, 75,* 134–141.

BIBLIOGRAPHY

Nursing Clinics of North America, Volume 29, No. 3, September 1994, is devoted to Community Health Nursing and Home Health Nursing. Most of the articles are from the perspective of the United States, however.

CHAPTER 22

Toward the Third Millennium: New Approaches to Nursing

Joyce J. Fitzpatrick

The third millennium is upon us . . .

To say that health care is in a state of transition is indeed an understatement. To say that health care is in a state of revolution is, conversely, an overstatement. Perhaps the most accurate descriptors of the "health" of the health care system are imbedded in the Chinese meanings underlying the term "crisis"—it is considered both a "threat" and an "opportunity for growth."

This chapter is concerned with the changes inherent in health care systems globally, with particular reference to the positioning necessary for relative stability in the third millennium, and with specific reference to the worldwide changes necessary for the professional discipline of nursing. Highlighted within the systems of health care are both primary health care and its subset of home care. Research and nursing education challenges for the future are identified, and a plea is made for enhancement of our international collaborations.

CURRENT STATUS OF NURSING WORLDWIDE

Never before has there been such consistency and increased communication among professional nurses throughout the world. Undoubtedly, some of these developments can be traced directly to the changes in our political, economic, and social interactions. Some of the communication is directly related to the technological developments that make it possible for all of us to communicate rapidly and travel quickly. The futurists among us have referred to this time as an "information age," when information is the medium of exchange and the source of power.

NURSING EDUCATION

Currently, consistency is developing in nursing education throughout the world. Efforts to enhance nursing education have been focused on strengthening both specialist and generalist education. Within generalist preparation for professional nursing, whether at the basic diploma level offered by hospitals and universities or the degree level offered by universities, there is a growing expansion of the focus on community-based models of care, including home care, public health, and primary care nursing. Within the generalist programs in nursing, there is a need for a stronger focus on public health. Advanced practice nurses, as the specialists in nursing, can now be found in a range of areas, including primary care, acute care, and long-term care. Although the term "advanced practice nursing" may be more characteristic of the model of education in the United States, there are similarities in specialty practice that are independent of the formal educational process throughout the world.

NURSING SCIENCE: THEORY DEVELOPMENT AND RESEARCH

Development of nursing knowledge has expanded considerably during the last 20 years, as nurses have become scientists and members of interdisciplinary research teams. Further, it can be expected that this knowledge development will continue to gain strength in this era of technological advancements. Particularly relevant is research related to the prevention, treatment, and cure of major diseases. Recently, we have witnessed a shift in health care research toward the social causes of poor health (e.g., lifestyle choices, poverty, and culture).

NURSING CLASSIFICATION SYSTEMS: DATA SETS

Recent developments include various national and international efforts to classify the professional "work" that nurses do and the outcomes of professional nursing interventions. Such classification systems include attention to the following components: nursing assessment; nursing diagnosis, nursing interventions, nurse-sensitive patient outcomes; and patient satisfaction.

PRIMARY HEALTH CARE

Primary health care has received considerable attention throughout our global discussions of health and health care delivery. Reference to primary health care can be found in many of the World Health Organization (WHO) discussions particularly since the Alma Alta Declaration (described later). A brief discussion of selected definitions of primary health care, with particular attention to the WHO definition and the recent U.S. Institute of Medicine definition follows.

WHO: Health for All by the Year 2000

In 1978, the term *primary health care* was first coined by WHO to describe a global strategy to view health as integral to social and economic relationships, and to create partnerships with communities to affect positive health changes. This Alma Alta Declaration, named after the geographic location within the Soviet Union where the conference occurred, quickly became known by the project goal: "Health for All by the Year 2000."

Institute of Medicine (IOM) Definition, 1994

The IOM Committee released a preliminary report in 1994. The following definition was included. Primary care is the provision of integrated, accessible health care services by clinicians who are accountable for addressing most personal health care needs, developing sustained partnerships with patients, and practicing within the context of family and community (IOM, 1994).

Various hallmarks of primary health care can be identified across definitions. These include care that is comprehensive, accessible, client centered, community based, and care that focuses on prevention of disease and promotion of health. Home care is an important subset of primary health care. Thus, the hallmarks of primary care delineated subsequently apply also to home care. They include the following:

Comprehensive care. Care that is holistic and responsive to the total range of situations and problems the patient presents

Accessible care. Care that is available to the patients/clients/persons that is both physically and psychologically within their reach

Client-centered care. Care that is directly related to the needs of the patient/client/person that is responsive to the problems and concerns that they present

Community-based care. Care that is delivered within community settings (e.g., local health centers, churches, schools, and importantly, the individual's home)

Prevention. Care that is focused at all times on the comprehensive prevention of illnesses, whether they are the primary presenting illnesses, related illnesses, or other new and unrelated problems

In general, then, definitions of primary care can be summarized as follows: Primary care is comprehensive; it includes primary, secondary, and tertiary prevention. Primary prevention includes health promotion and prevention of illness.

PRIMARY CARE RESEARCH

Primary care research is focused on the effectiveness of health care practices, cost of care, access to care, and quality of care. Various priorities have been identified for the research on primary care. Because of the complexities of the questions imbedded in the research initiatives, health scientists will continue to address these issues well into the 21st century. These priorities include the following:

- Effectiveness and costs of primary care
- Relationships between cost and quality as a function of access

- Organization of practitioners
- Community-based programs
- International comparisons

HOME CARE

Home care, the particular focus of this book, together with public health nursing and primary health care, forms an integral core of the health care system of the future. We recently have witnessed a rapid movement of delivery of primary care, acute care, and long-term care into home care settings, bringing new challenges for education, practice, and research. As is demonstrated in this book, these challenges are many. It is our hope that the most positive outcome of this book would be the collective wisdom and knowledge of current advances in home care delivery, knowledge that we all might use in our individual projects and communities.

Health care of the future in the United States will reflect many of these changes.

Revitalization of public health system. Concomitant with a focus on prevention and health promotion, it is imperative that we redesign our public health systems, so that they are both more extensive and more comprehensive.

Decentralized public health system. Health care must be controlled at the local source of power. There are numerous examples of inefficient systems of health care delivery that are too far removed from the people they serve. A public health system should develop a unified, coherent health care policy to promote national and international health care goals.

Delivery networks close to work and home. Not only should the source of control reside close to the recipients, but also the actual health centers or clinics should be located in the individual's community, close to work and close to home.

Technology supplements to traditional care. A wide range of technology continues to be developed to extend diagnosis and treatment in health care delivery. We can anticipate that these technological developments will multiply.

Health information and self-care models. As discussed later, we can anticipate a greater diffusion of health information to the general public, through the extensions of computer networks and information systems. Further, a model of consumer empowerment will extend the demand for personal health information.

In summary, several changes in society call for teamwork in the delivery of primary health care of the future. These include the following:

1. Changes in the concept of health care—from a focus solely on disease and death to one on health and well-being
2. Changes in the models of medical practice and nursing practice
3. Changes in the locus of health service delivery—from hospitals and outpatient departments to neighborhood-based, ambulatory, health care centers
4. Changes in the status of the patient—from passive recipients to active participants in the care process
5. Changes in relationships among health professionals—from traditional, authoritarian, status-oriented, hierarchical relationships to more democratic, participatory, peer relationships
6. Changes in the financing of health care services

CHALLENGES

Research

As we proceed to design delivery systems for the future, it is equally imperative that we construct research to evaluate the outcomes of our new delivery systems. Several factors require our attention including the following:

Global perspectives. In a world of fluid geographic and national boundaries, it is important that we consider the global implications of our projects and findings.

Population-based research initiatives. Epidemiological approaches to research and evaluation will be central to projects of the future, as we try to address the greater social and economical good.

Enhanced public-private partnerships. Throughout the world, partnerships will be key to our health care future, partnerships that are reflected in education, practice, and research.

Nursing Education

Although we have targeted nursing challenges for this book, these same challenges are relevant to all health care professions. They include the following components:

- Interdisciplinary health care education
- Distance learning programs
- Technology enhancements
- Continuing education and lifelong professional learning

International Collaboration

Three aspects of international collaboration are highlighted here; they are presented as facets of the potential forms of collaboration, not as an inclusive list of components. These examples include multicultural research, formal collaborative relationships between institutions, and faculty and student exchange programs.

Public Education

Concomitant with the paradigm shift to a consumer-driven model of health care is the need to focus on public education about health care. Three aspects of public education will be highlighted: health awareness information, self-help programs, and media information. Health professionals, both within their provider roles and as consumers themselves, need to be actively involved in the direction of this paradigm shift.

Health Awareness Information

Ask your neighbors what they know about common indicators of their own health. Do they know generally that "exercise is good," or specifically the heart rate induced by exercise that is most beneficial to cardiovascular fitness and overall health? How could anyone continue to smoke when faced with the overwhelming evidence that directly links prolonged tobacco smoking to negative health consequences? Is nutrition just for nutritionists and dietitians to understand, or is it of relevance to public health and, therefore, the individual consumer's health?

Self-Help Programs

Often the most understanding and supportive persons are those who have experienced similar events. Self-help groups function as support groups, assisting the persons, healthy or ill, to derive meaning from their current experience, and to take control of their own life and health. Self-help groups may have religious or spiritual connections, cultural or social connections, or may be solely based on an illness condition. In a land that prides itself on "rugged individualism," such as the United States, self-help groups often are focused on helping the individual overcome the disease.

Media Information

As health professionals, we have a powerful tool that is often under-used in our public health initiatives and our public awareness programs. Journalists for newspapers, magazines, and radio and television programs could be provided with health information that informs the public and ultimately improves the health of the public. Knowledge is power. The first step to gain control over one's health is to gain the necessary knowledge.

CONCLUSION

In conclusion, our challenges for the next millennium are not ones that are beyond our comprehension. Rather, they directly flow from our understanding of the current and immediate future changes within our health care delivery system. The only challenge we face is the turning point described by the Chinese translation of crisis, the fork in the road that leads us to a threat or an opportunity for growth.

REFERENCE

Institute of Medicine. (1994). *Defining primary care: An interim report.* Washington, DC: National Academy Press.

Index